THE MANAGEMENT OF NUTRITIONAL EMERGENCIES IN LARGE POPULATIONS

C. DE VILLE DE GOYET

*Research Centre in Disaster Epidemiology,
Catholic University of Louvain,
Belgium*

J. SEAMAN

*London Technical Group,
United Kingdom*

and

U. GEIJER

Swedish Red Cross Society

UNITED NATIONS

WORLD HEALTH ORGANIZATION

GENEVA

1978

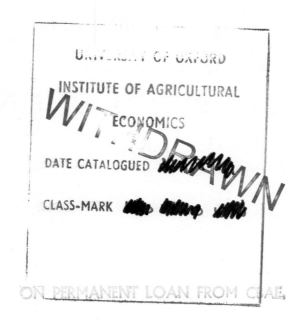
ISBN 92 4 154131 8

PRINTED IN SWITZERLAND

CONTENTS

6

Preface

This guide is intended for use by health personnel responsible for the field management of nutritional emergencies in populations, namely, the medical or allied personnel from national or provincial health services or from relief agencies in the country affected.

It is particularly concerned with severe nutritional emergencies, that is, mass starvation caused by the interruption of food supplies to the population over a long period. Unusual food shortages may be caused by major crop failures, war and civil conflicts, or natural disasters. Relief personnel responsible for short-term food distribution following a major disaster such as an earthquake or cyclone may also find these guidelines useful, although they were specifically prepared for the management of situations in which populations suffer from widespread and severe malnutrition.

No mention is made of social, cultural, or political factors that are critical during famines, nor of rehabilitation. The guide is concerned, as it were, with fire-fighting rather than fire prevention or reconstruction.

No short booklet can provide guidelines applicable to each and every situation. Adaptation and improvisation will be necessary to some extent. All the examples given are based on experience, and it is hoped that they will be helpful in the preparation of local procedures and guides for the on-site training of relief workers in each country.

ACKNOWLEDGEMENTS AND REFERENCES

Acknowledgement is due to many individuals both in and outside WHO for their valuable advice and criticism based upon long experience of field work.   The authors are also grateful to the League of Red Cross Societies, the Catholic Relief Services, and Oxfam for their valuable assistance in the preparation of this guide.

Material and ideas have been drawn from many sources, but particularly from the following publications:

Guide to food and health relief operations in disasters.   New York, Protein-Calorie Advisory Group (PAG) of the United Nations System, 1977.

BLIX, G., HOFVANDER, Y. & VAHLQUIST, V., ed.   *Famine: a symposium dealing with nutrition and relief operations in times of disaster.*   Uppsala, Almqvist & Wikell for Swedish Nutrition Foundation and Swedish International Development Authority, 1971.

KING, M.H. *Nutrition for developing countries.*   Nairobi, Oxford University Press, 1972.

Food emergency manual.   Rome, World Food Programme (new edition in preparation).

CAMERON, M. & HOFVANDER, Y.   *Manual on feeding infants and young children.*   2nd edition, New York, Protein-Calorie Advisory Group of the United Nations System, 1976.

A debt of gratitude is also owed to the Literary Executor of the late Sir Ronald A. Fisher, F.R.S., to Dr Frank Yates, F.R.S., and to Longman Group Ltd, London, for permission to reprint Table A in Annex 6 from their book *Statistical Tables for Biological, Agricultural and Medical Research* (6th edition, 1974).

1. Normal and emergency needs

Basic facts about food and nutrition are given in Annex 1, which should be consulted by readers who are not thoroughly familiar with nutritional concepts. Energy and protein requirements in normal and emergency situations are briefly summarized below.[1]

Normal situations

Recommended intakes

The energy and protein intakes considered as safe by WHO/FAO for each age group and physiological condition[2] are shown in Annex 1.

Vulnerable groups

The energy and protein requirements of women are increased during pregnancy—by +1.5 MJ (350 kcal$_{th}$) and +15 g protein per day—and during lactation—by +2.3 MJ (550 kcal$_{th}$) and +20 g protein per day—over and above their normal requirements.

Preschool children (0–5 years) require proportionally more energy and protein for each kg of body weight than adults. They are more vulnerable to malnutrition.

Emergency situations

The WHO/FAO safe intakes of energy and protein[2] have not yet been attained by the majority of people in developing countries. In nutritional emergencies caused by food shortage, relief planning based on these standards is unrealistic. The maintenance of energy intake at a level adequate for survival must be the primary consideration.

---

[1] Energy values are expressed in the SI unit, the megajoule (MJ). The equivalents in the superseded unit, the thermochemical kilocalorie (kcal$_{th}$) are given in parentheses. 1 MJ = 239 kcal$_{th}$. 1000 kcal$_{th}$ = 4.184 MJ.

[2] PASSMORE, R. ET AL. *Handbook on human nutritional requirements*, Geneva, World Health Organization, 1974 (Monograph Series, No. 61).

Table 1 shows the minimum amount of energy required to sustain life.

TABLE 1. EMERGENCY ENERGY INTAKE PER PERSON [a]

Group	Height (cm)	Emergency subsistence (for a few weeks) MJ (kcal$_{th}$) per day	Temporary maintenance (for many months) MJ (kcal$_{th}$) per day
0–1 years[b]	under 75	3.4 (800)	3.4 (800)
1–3 years	75– 96	4.6 (1 100)	5.4 (1 300)
4–6 years	96–117	5.4 (1 300)	6.7 (1 600)
7–9 years	117–136	6.3 (1 500)	7.5 (1 800)
10 years or over:	over 136		
male		7.1 (1 700)	8.4 (2 000)
female		6.3 (1 500)	7.5 (1 800)
Pregnant or lactating women		8.0 (1 900)	9.2 (2 200)
Average per day per person		about 6.3 MJ (1 500 kcal$_{th}$)	about 7.5 MJ (1 800 kcal$_{th}$)

[a] Adapted from Mayer, J. Famine relief: what kind of organization and what types of trained personnel are needed in the field. In: Blix, G. et al. *Famine: a symposium...*, Uppsala, 1971.
[b] Levels for infants are similar to those recommended for normal situation.

The emergency subsistence level is the estimated level below which large-scale starvation and death should be expected if the population is of normal body size and is required to perform some work.

A prolonged maintenance diet at the level indicated above is likely to result in some loss of body weight. Supplementary feeding of vulnerable groups is essential to provide extra energy and nutrients.

Even under "normal conditions", without any emergency, the energy intake of some populations is comparable to or less than the temporary maintenance level—7.5 MJ (1800 kcal$_{th}$). When resources are scarce, it may not be justifiable to provide this amount to some segments of the population, and a level as low as 6.3 MJ (1500 kcal$_{th}$) will have to be maintained for extended periods. The decision will depend on local conditions.

2. Major deficiency diseases in emergencies

- **Protein-energy malnutrition** (PEM) is the most important health problem during a nutritional emergency.
  Severe PEM can present several forms:
  - *Nutritional marasmus* is characterized by a severe wasting away of fat and muscle ("skin and bone"). It is the commonest form in most nutritional emergencies.
  - *Kwashiorkor* is characterized by oedema, usually starting at the lower extremities.
  - *Marasmic kwashiorkor* is a combination of wasting and oedema. The treatment of severe forms of PEM is presented in Chapter 5.

- **Mineral and vitamin deficiencies** may also be important.
  - *Severe anemia* is common and requires a daily intake of iron for an extended period of time.
  - *Vitamin A deficiency,* the most important vitamin deficiency, is characterized by night blindness and/or eye lesions which may lead to permanent total blindness. The severe forms are usually associated with PEM.
  - Other deficiency conditions are less common: beriberi, pellagra, scurvy, rickets.
  - Mineral and vitamin deficiencies must be identified and the individuals affected or at risk treated by administration of the missing nutrient.

Protein-energy malnutrition (PEM)

Protein-energy malnutrition is a problem in many developing countries, even in normal times. Most commonly it affects children between the ages of 6 months and 5 years (especially around 18–24 months), i.e., at the time when they are most vulnerable to the common infectious diseases such as gastroenteritis and measles. PEM may simply be due to shortage of food, or it may be precipitated by lack of appetite and an increase in nutrient requirements and losses caused by infection.

Chronic PEM has many short- and long-term physical and mental effects, including growth retardation, a malnourished child being lighter and shorter than a better-fed child of the same age.

In times of nutritional emergency it is primarily the more acute forms of PEM that have to be dealt with. These are characterized by a rapid loss of weight and may be evident in a much wider range of age groups than usual. For example, significant numbers of older children, adolescents, and adults may also be affected.

Past experience has shown that many emergencies affect the supply of food to only a proportion of the population concerned. The situation will obviously vary from place to place, but it is often the case that only a small proportion of the total population presents clinical signs of severe PEM. For each case of severe clinical PEM there may well be 10 moderate cases and 100 children of "near normal" nutritional status. Progression from moderate to clinically severe forms is rapid.

Severe forms of PEM [1]

The severe forms of PEM are:

> nutritional marasmus
> kwashiorkor
> marasmic kwashiorkor

Nutritional marasmus results from prolonged starvation (see Fig. 1).

The main sign is a severe wasting away of fat and muscle. The child is very thin ("skin and bone"), most of the fat and muscle mass having been expended to provide energy. It is the most frequent form of PEM in cases of severe food shortage.

---

[1] For treatment, see Chapter 5.

Associated signs can be:

- A thin "old man" face.

- "Baggy pants" (the loose skin of a child's buttocks hanging down).

- The children concerned are usually active and may appear to be very alert in spite of their condition.

- There is no oedema (swelling that pits on pressure) of the lower extremities.

FIG. 1. CHILD SUFFERING FROM NUTRITIONAL MARASMUS

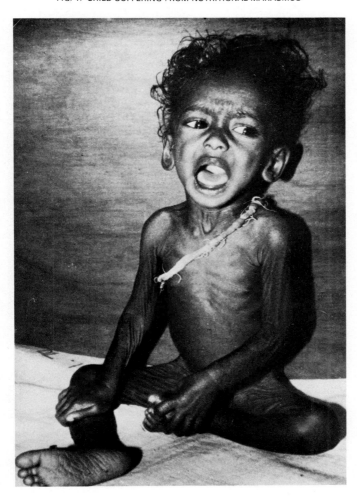

Kwashiorkor (see Fig. 2 and Fig. 3). The main sign is oedema, usually starting at the lower extremities and extending, in more advanced cases, to the arms and face. Oedema may be detected by the production of a definite pit in the pretibial region as a result of moderate pressure for three seconds with the thumb over the lower end of the tibia.

The child may look "fat" so that the parents regard him as well-fed.

Associated signs can be:

● Hair changes: loss of pigmentation, curly hair becomes straight (an African child may appear to have much longer hair), easy pluckability (the hair comes out easily with a very gentle pull).

FIG. 2. A SEVERE CASE OF KWASHIORKOR SHOWING OEDEMA
AND SKIN AND HAIR CHANGES

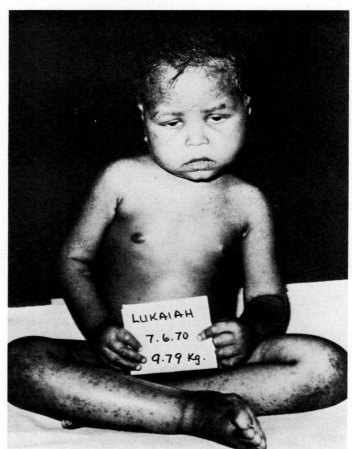

WORLD HEALTH ORGANIZATION

THE MANAGEMENT OF NUTRITIONAL EMERGENCIES IN LARGE POPULATIONS

by

C. DE VILLE DE GOYET, J. SEAMAN & U. GEIJER

CORRIGENDA

Page 16, footnote 1

Delete:

[1] UNICEF tablets specified as containing 0.2 g dried iron sulfate (equivalent to 368 mg of elemental iron) and 250 µg of folate are recommended for routine use— UNIPAC catalogue number 15 500 10 (bottles of 1000 tablets).

Insert:

[1] UNICEF tablets containing 300 mg of ferrous sulfate ($FeSo_4.7H_2O$), or about 60 mg of elemental iron, and 250 µg of folate are recommended for routine use— UNIPAC catalogue number 15 500 10 (bottles of 1000 tablets).

Page 20, Table 2, right-hand column, second entry (Xerophthalmia)

Delete: intramuscular injection of 55 000 µg water-miscible retinol palmitate (100 000 IU of vitamin A) followed the next day by oral administration of 110 000 µg (200 000 IU of vitamin A) ; adequate protein intake is essential

Insert: intramuscular injection of 55 000 µg water-miscible retinol palmitate (100 000 IU of vitamin A) followed the next day by oral administration of 68 000 µg of retinol acetate or 110 000 µg of retinol palmitate (200 000 IU of vitamin A) ; adequate protein intake is essential

- Skin lesions and depigmentation: dark skin may become lighter in some places, especially in the skin folds; skin may peel off (especially on the legs), and ulceration may occur.   The skin lesions may look very like burns.
- Children with kwashiorkor are usually apathetic and miserable and show no signs of hunger.   It is difficult to persuade then to eat.

The associated signs of kwashiorkor do not always occur.   In some cases oedema may be the only visible sign, in others all the associated signs may be present.

Marasmic kwashiorkor.   This is a mixed form with oedema occurring in children who are otherwise marasmic and who may or may not have the other associated signs of kwashiorkor.

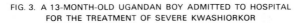

FIG. 3. A 13-MONTH-OLD UGANDAN BOY ADMITTED TO HOSPITAL
FOR THE TREATMENT OF SEVERE KWASHIORKOR

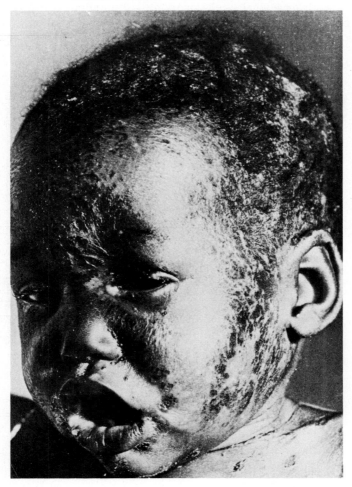

Specific deficencies

While severe PEM is usually the most important health problem during a nutritional emergency, mineral and vitamin deficiencies may also be important. Their treatment is summarized in Table 2.

Anaemia

Nearly all malnourished children are anaemic as a result of iron deficiency and often of folic acid deficiency. Moderate or severe anaemia is diagnosed by pulling down the lower eyelid and looking for pallor of the conjunctiva. The causes are generally multiple (nutritional deficiencies, e.g., of iron and folic acid, malaria, hookworm infestation, etc.). Treatment of moderate forms consists of the daily administration of iron and folic acid for several weeks or months throughout recovery. Supervision of treatment can be difficult under emergency conditions. The daily dose is 100–150 mg of iron with 100 μg of folic acid.[1] Malaria and hook-

FIG. 4. XEROPHTHALMIA IS DIFFICULT TO DETECT AND CHILDREN
ARE OFTEN BROUGHT TO HOSPITAL MUCH TOO LATE TO SAVE THEIR EYES

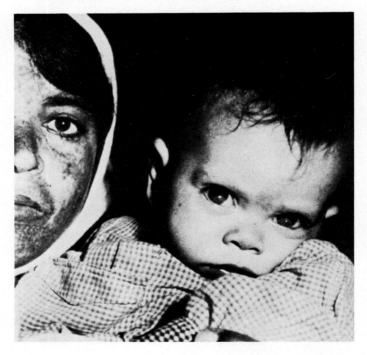

---

[1] UNICEF tablets specified as containing 0.2 g dried iron sulfate (equivalent to 368 mg of elemental iron) and 250 μg of folate are recommended for routine use—UNIPAC catalogue number 15 500 10 (bottles of 1000 tablets).

worm infestation should be treated and children (and perhaps women) need to receive additional food for faster recovery. Very severe anaemia (extreme pallor, white mucous membranes, difficulty in breathing) should be referred to medical facilities for blood transfusion where possible.

Vitamin A deficiency and xerophthalmia [1]

Vitamin A deficiency is the leading cause of permanent blindness in preschool children. It is almost always associated with some degree of protein-energy malnutrition. Xerophthalmia is the term used to describe the eye signs caused by vitamin A deficiency (see Fig. 4). The daily requirement of retinol rises from 300 μg for an infant to 750 μg for an adult and 1200 μg for a pregnant woman. If the vitamin A is provided by vegetable foods (carotenes) and not by animal products (which includes full cream milk) the amount should be multiplied by six, i.e., range from 1800 μg to 7200 μg (average: about 4000 μg per day per person).

Vitamin A deficiency is most likely to be a problem in areas where the diets of the very poor, even in normal times, do not meet requirements. Since most vitamin A is derived from vegetable sources (green vegetables, most yellow fruits and vegetables, e.g., mangoes, papayas, and carrots, red palm oil, etc.) and these are, in many countries, only seasonally available, there may be a higher incidence of xerophthalmia towards the end of the dry season, when liver stores of the vitamin are depleted.

Since vitamin A is stored in the liver, a sudden deterioration in the diet does not necessarily produce an immediate sharp rise in the incidence of cases, and there may well be a delay of several months until vitamin A deficiency occurs.

Symptoms. One of the first symptoms of vitamin A deficiency is night blindness. Those affected are unable to see at low light intensities e.g., after sunset or inside a hut) when normal individuals can still see reasonably well.

This symptom is difficult to confirm in small children, but there may be a local word for it and mothers may recognize that the night vision of their children is impaired. Indeed, the existence of a local word should be taken as suggesting at least a potential problem.

The following eye lesions are caused by vitamin A deficiency:

— areas on the conjunctiva which become dry, opaque, and dull (xerosis [2])
— accumulation (often triangular in shape) of foamy material on the conjunctiva, usually towards the outer side of the iris (Bitot's spots [2])
— the cornea becomes dry and dull (corneal xerosis), and this may be followed by the most severe signs, namely, clouding, ulceration, and

---

[1] See also: SOMMER, A. *Field guide to detection and control of xerophthalmia,* Geneva, World Health Organization, 1978.

[2] Slight degrees of xerosis and Bitot's spots may be stained by the application of a small drop of lissamine green or rose bengal 1 % solution with a 10 μl Eppendorf pipette. See: SAUTER, J.J. *Trop. Doc.,* **6**: 91-93 (1976).

(even within the space of a few hours) perforation of the cornea, leading to loss of eye contents and permanent blidness. Ulceration and perforation may occur with alarming rapidity, especially in young children who are suffering from measles or some other acute febrile illness.

The presence of any of these signs in even a few children indicates that many more children are at risk.

Prevention. The best way to prevent xerophthalmia is to provide suffi-cient carotenes or vitamin A in the diet. Note that vitamin A is removed from dried skim milk (DSM) with the fat during processing. Some DSM is supplemented in the factory (e.g., milk provided by UNICEF, WFP, or EEC). This should be indicated on the package and is an important fact to check.

In high-risk areas it may be necessary to administer a high dose of vita-min A periodically to every child, lactating mother, and woman pregnant for more than 6 months. This should be seriously considered if:

— the diet is grossly deficient in vitamin A;

— more than 2% of children under 5 years of age have conjunctival xero-sis including Bitot's spots;

— old corneal lesions (scars) are found in one or more children in every 1000.

A single UNICEF soluble capsule containing 110 000 μg of retinol pal-mitate (200 000 IU of vitamin A) will provide protection for 4–6 months. It should be repeated at an interval of 4 months. Half a dose should be given to children under 1 year. Administration of vitamin A should be recorded on the child's ration card. Overdosage (indicated by headache, vomiting, etc.) is exceptional and may be caused by too frequent (e.g., daily) administration of a high dose.

Vitamin B1 deficiency (beriberi)

The problem of vitamin B1 or thiamine deficiency is less common and is confined to certain areas, e.g., those where the diet is of white polished rice or where people have had to live exclusively on a starchy staple food such as cassava. Several forms exist:

● the "dry" form with neuritis leading to paralysis of the limbs;
● the "wet" form with acute swelling of the body (oedema) and other signs of cardiac failure, leading to sudden death (especially among infants);
● the moderate form, which can be very common, characterized by loss of appetite, malaise, and severe weakness, especially in the legs. These signs may last for many months.

An average intake of approximately 1 mg thiamine daily is sufficient to prevent beriberi; sources are undermilled cereals, legumes, green leaves, etc. Parboiling of rice should be encouraged. Rice for camp use should not be too polished.

Niacin deficiency (pellagra)

Pellagra is characterized by a bilaterally symmetrical skin rash found only on those surfaces of the body exposed to sunlight. It is often marked by severe diarrhoea and mental deterioration.

This deficiency is found mostly among maize- and sorghum-eating populations and is prevented by an average intake of 15–20 mg of niacin per day per person. Sources are legumes and cereals (undermilled).

Vitamin C deficiency (scurvy)

Scurvy is easily recognized: the gums are swollen, particularly between the teeth, and bleed easily. The big joints (knee, hip, etc.) may also appear swollen, although bleeding can take place in any tissue. Haemorrhages on the surface of the bone (subperiosteal) are painful and can cause a pseudo-paralysis in infants. Scurvy can be prevented by providing at least 10 mg daily of ascorbic acid (vitamin C)—i.e., 15 ml of citrus juice, one quarter of an orange, a small tomato, or 20 g of leafy vegetables. If gum swelling does not respond to vitamin C, the cause is not scurvy but poor mouth hygiene.

Vitamin D deficiency (rickets)

Rickets is characterized by deformed, soft bones. The skull has an irregular square form with bossing, while the long bones are bowed with enlarged extremities. Walking is delayed. The best way to prevent rickets is by exposing the unclothed body of the child to sunlight.

Specific deficiencies and nutritional relief

The distribution of multivitamin tablets to the entire population of the affected area is a waste of time and money. The best means of providing vitamins is an adequate diet. Most multivitamin preparations contain only very small quantities of individual vitamins and must be taken at least daily to be of any use. The following approach to the problem of vitamin deficiencies should be adopted:

1. *Identify the deficiencies of public health importance.* For instance, is xerophthalmia a potential problem? Is scurvy or beriberi to be reasonably expected? Such questions are best answered by:

— evaluating the respective intakes of major vitamins in the actual diet,

— initiating a surveillance system (see Chapter 3).

2. Should an obvious dietary deficiency be identified or the presence of typical signs of a specific clinical deficiency be reported and confirmed, *the diet should be corrected by providing foods rich in the missing vitamins and/or minerals.*

3. Should this be impossible or insufficient, mass administration of the *specific* vitamin is indicated. It should be given in adequate quantities.

TABLE 2. CURATIVE TREATMENT OF SPECIFIC DEFICIENCIES (IN BRIEF)

What	When	How much and how long
Moderate to severe anaemia	● marked pallor of conjunctiva	100–200 mg of iron with 100 μg of folic acid daily in 2 or 3 divided doses several weeks or months until recovery
Xerophthalmia	● night blindness ● any ocular sign of vitamin A deficiency ● severe PEM	intramuscular injection of 55 000 μg water-miscible retinol palmitate (100 000 IU of vitamin A) followed the next day by oral administration of 110 000 μg (200 000 IU of vitamin A; adequate protein intake is essential
Beriberi	● any suspicion of vitamin B 1 deficiency	50 mg of thiamine followed by 10 mg daily until recovery
Pellagra	● any suspicion of niacin deficiency	300 mg of niacin per mouth daily until recovery (usually a few days in acute cases)
Scurvy	● any haemorrhagic symptom in a malnourished child	500 mg or more ascorbic acid daily until recovery
Rickets	● any suspect bone deformation in young child	no more than 100 000–300 000 IU (2.5–7.5 mg) of colecalciferol (vitamin D) in a single dose or 1 000 IU (25 μg) daily for 10–30 days; [a] exposure of the skin to sunlight.

[a] An overdose of colecalciferol is dangerous.

3. Assessment and surveillance of nutritional status

Suitable methods must be adopted for the rapid and objective measurement of the nutritional status:

- of individuals eligible for special food relief (individual screening);
- of communities, in order to detect changes with time and decide priorities in food distribution (nutritional surveillance).

Weight-for-height is the best indicator for the diagnosis of nutritional status, nutritional surveillance, and individual screening. Weight-for-age and arm circumference are less reliable for assessment and screening but can be used to measure changes with time. Oedema rates are a valuable indicator when kwashiorkor is the prevalent form of PEM in the area.

Results of surveys and surveillance must be interpreted with caution. They can be misleading unless the individuals measured are representative of the whole population and the technique is standardized and properly used.

Why measure malnutrition in emergencies?

During a nutritional emergency, the relief foods may be scarce and should be given to the people in greatest need. Since much of a population may be able to supply part or all of its own food, it is very useful to have an objective and quantifiable measure of nutritional status.

Measurement of nutritional status in emergencies relies mainly upon taking body measurements (anthropometry), particularly height, weight, and arm circumference. Valuable information may also be obtained from simpler methods, for example, monitoring clinic records or measuring the prevalence of oedema.

The commonest reasons for measuring malnutrition in a relief programme are:

Initial assessment.   A rapid survey of the population should be done before initiating a relief programme, in order to identify the areas or groups that are most
affected.   Surveys of this type need to be carefully designed and conducted by an
experienced team.   They will not be considered further.[1]

Individual screening.   Body measurements may be used to select the malnourished individuals eligible for food relief for themselves or their whole family.

Nutritional surveillance of the population.   The repeated measuring of entire
communities gives an idea of differences among the various population groups and
changes in nutritional status with time.   It may be used to decide priorities in the
distribution of relief and will also provide some information about the effectiveness
of the relief programme.   In nutritional surveillance one is not interested in monitoring the progress of a child, but in knowing whether the overall nutritional condition of *village (or camp) A* is good or bad, is better or worse than that of village B and
C (and so requires more supplies and personnel), and whether it is improving or
deteriorating with time.   Nutritional surveillance should not be confused with the
"surveillance" or follow-up of an *individual* child in nutrition centres or health services.

Indicators of malnutrition

Clinical signs of PEM or specific deficiencies

Clinical signs in this context are signs that can be rapidly assessed by
touching or examining the child concerned rather than by instruments or
tests.

● *Oedema.*   In extreme situations or where kwashiorkor is the prevalent type of malnutrition, simple surveys (or screening) for this sign may
be sufficiently precise, without using body measurements (anthropometry).   According to the local situation, oedema of the feet can be looked
for in young children, lactating women, and possibly older people.

● *Clinical marasmus* (if a standard clinical definition is used).

● *Night blindness* (mothers should be questioned), *eye signs* of xerophthalmia (vitamin A deficiency).

● *Selected clinical signs* indicative of other vitamin or mineral (iron,
etc.) deficiency of potential local importance, depending on the basic diet
of the population.

In very severe famine with widespread advanced starvation, clinical
signs are most useful as indicators and may be temporarily sufficient when
resources are limited.   The main problem lies in the fact that observations
by different persons are not easily comparable and can hardly be standardized.

---

[1] Interested readers are referred to: *Guide to food and health relief operations in disasters.*
New York, Protein-Calorie Advisory Group of the United Nations System, 1977.

Body measurements

Body measurements are used to detect malnutrition, but not food shortage, since malnutrition can also be caused by ignorance or faulty feeding habits in the presence of sufficient food. The results of body measurements can be misleading if considered in isolation.

Chronic undernutrition leads to a slowing in a child's rate of growth. A chronically malnourished child will be short for his age ("stunted") although he may be of otherwise normal proportions.

An *acute* episode of severe undernutrition results in a loss of muscle and fat which are used up to provide energy, and the individual becomes thinner without significant effect upon height ("wasting").

In an emergency what is important is the measurement of *acute* malnutrition, the effects of chronic malnutrition being of less concern. Because *both* stunting *and* wasting result in low weight-for-*age*, relating body measurements to age is not recommended. Two measurements are commonly used to assess acute malnutrition ("wasting"):

Weight-for-height. Here a child's weight is compared with the height of a "reference" (well-nourished) child of the same height. Results are expressed as "percentages of reference", e.g., 80% of standard weight-for-height or in relation to (above or below) a pre-selected cut-off point.[1]

Arm circumference (AC). Well-nourished children have a nearly constant arm circumference (about 16 cm) between 1 and 5 years. Undernourished children have a thinner upper arm and a smaller AC. Children can be classified as malnourished if their AC falls below an arbitrarily specified level. If ages are not known, AC can be related to height (arm-circumference-for-height).

Presence of diseases associated with PEM

These include measles, diarrhoea (defined for instance as three or more loose stools per day), whooping cough, etc.

Mortality data

PEM is associated with increased mortality among young children (e.g., from measles, etc.).

The data collected should be expressed as rates; for example, the rate per thousand of marasmus among infants (aged 0–1) in a refugee camp is:

$$\frac{\text{number of infants with marasmus in the camp}}{\text{total number of infants in the camp}} \times 1000$$

---

[1]Cut-off points at 2 or 3 standard deviations below the median reference values were recently recommended (See Annex 3).

Body measurements

N.B. A very great effort should be made to measure children accurately. Small errors (e.g., 2–3 cm in height) in the measurement of a younger child may lead to significant errors in the classification of the child's nutritional status.

Select only one indicator:

● Weight-for-height, the recommended body measurement in times of emergency, is a sensitive indicator of acute malnutrition. It is fairly independent of sex, race, and age (up to about 10 years of age). It requires a sufficient number of robust scales and adequate training of personnel. Neither condition is easy to meet in an acute emergency situation.

● If ages are not known, arm-circumference-for-height is the best alternative. Measuring arm circumference instead of weight results in only a marginal saving of time compared to that required for travelling and assembling people. Several techniques such as the QUAC stick (Annex 5) have been devised to simplify field work and are useful for the screening of large numbers of children.

● As a second alternative, measurement of arm circumference alone (without measurement of height) is acceptable in situations where resources are extremely limited. Considerable time is saved by not measuring height. The sensitivity of the measurement as an indicator is poor but is sufficient in situations where PEM is severe and widespread.

Techniques

(*a*) *Weight measurement*

● Check the scales daily with the *same* known weight (e.g., a piece of metal), having first set the scale at zero.

● Remove the child's shoes and at least *heavy* clothing (a standard routine should be followed). Infants can be weighed without clothing to give more accurate readings.

● If a beam balance with a tray is used, make sure that the child sits properly and is not holding his mother or the static part of the scales. Beam scales should lie on a stable and horizontal surface (e.g., a wide board or a table).

● Read weight to nearest 100 g.

Various types of scales can be used in field conditions. For example:

— UNICEF standard beam balance: accurate, robust, for fixed centres. Frequent transportation on rough roads is not recommended.
— Healthometer (Continental Scale Corporation, USA): a beam balance, accurate and robust, suitable for use by mobile teams.

— Portable Salter scale (CMS Weighing Equipment, Ltd, England): the child is suspended from the scale which is hung from a branch or a tripod. Special "pants" are used to weigh babies (Fig. 5). Robust, cheap, and easy to carry, these scales should be replaced after one year because of stretching of the spring and inaccurate readings. The model with readings up to 25 kg ($\times$ 100 g) is recommended.

— Bar scales with platforms have been used in fixed centres. Their use requires training and caution. They may be too bulky and heavy for use by mobile teams.

— The Homs beam balance scale which is sturdy, accurate, and relatively easy to carry in a small car. It can be used for all age groups.

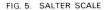

FIG. 5. SALTER SCALE

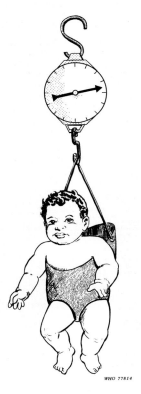

WHO 77814

Bathroom scales are not recommended.

Most types of scales (especially beam scales) are sensitive to dust and mud.

(b) Height measurement

Use a baby-board (see Fig. 6) for children unable to stand up (under 2 years or less than 85 cm).   Children should be quiet, relaxed (having a parent hold the child usually helps), and lying straight.   Gentle pressure should be applied upon both knees with one hand and care taken to see that the slide is in contact with the whole surface of the soles of the child's feet, not just the toes.   Measure to 1 cm (round off to the nearest cm: e.g., 90.0–90.4 cm = 90 cm, 90.5–90.9 cm = 91 cm).

When an upright measure is used the subject's heels should be together and touch the base of the upright, and the buttocks, the back of the heels, and the upper back should be in contact with the measuring stick (which can be locally made).   Measurement is to the highest point of the head when the child is looking straight ahead.   Shoes should be removed.   On average, children are about 1 cm shorter when standing up than when lying down.

FIG. 6.   USING A BABY-BOARD TO MEASURE A CHILD

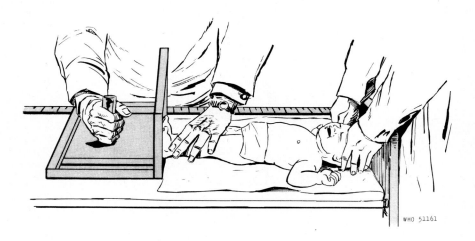

WHO 51161

(c) Arm-circumference measurement

The circumference is measured on the left upper arm *half way* between the end of the shoulder (acromion) and the tip of the elbow (olecranon). To locate this point, the arm is flexed at a right angle.   Then the arm is allowed to hang freely and a tape-measure (preferably of fibreglass) put firmly round it.   Do not pull too tight (Fig. 7).

FIG. 7.   MEASURING ARM CIRCUMFERENCE

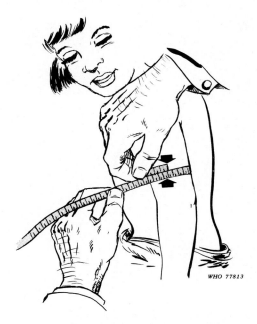

WHO 77813

Tapes or strips can be made locally from thin cardboard or X-ray films which are marked off in centimetres.[1] Special plastic tapes (insertion tapes) have been manufactured (Fig. 8).

Bangles, worn as arm ornaments in some countries, can be used for a rough screening of severely malnourished children.   A bangle of standard diameter is passed up the arm in one straight push.   If it goes above the elbow, the arm cir-

FIG. 8. INSERTION TAPE

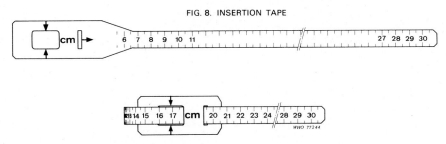

WHO 77244

From: Zerfas, A. J. *Am. J. clin. Nutr.*, **28**: 782–787 (1975).

---

[1] The cardboard tape or strips, X-ray films, or 8-mm cine films can be coloured according to the classification of the reading. (The X-ray film should first be scratched with a sharp point and then coloured with a spirit-based felt-tipped pen not quite up to the scratch line. Cut the film into 1-cm strips with scissors. About 40 strips can be made from one large X-ray film.)

FIG. 9. NUTRITIONAL STATUS CHART[a]

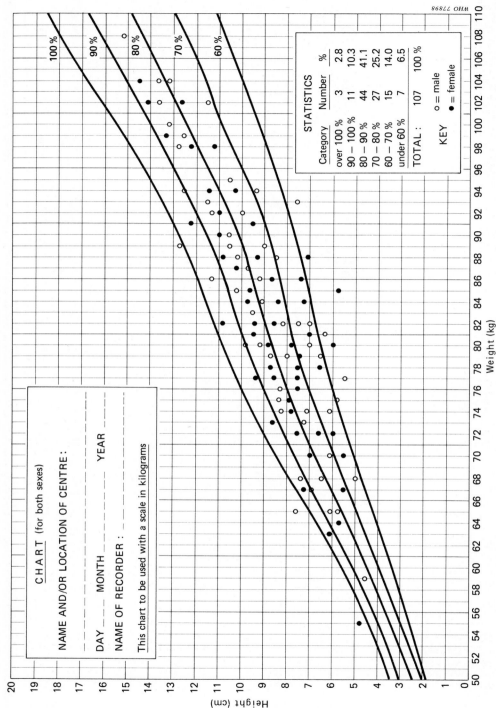

[a] Adapted from: CAPONE, C. A growth surveillance system for food and nutrition programs. In: *Integrating Title II program with locally operated nutrition, socio-economic and humanitarian activities*. Catholic Relief Services, 1977 (mimeographed).

The basic data are the same as those used by WHO for a forthcoming publication which gives specifications for a model growth chart. The measurements for children being screened are cumference is too small and the child is regarded as malnourished.   A bangle 4.0 cm in diameter passes up arms that are up to about 13.2 cm in circumference (the measurable circumference depends on the flexibility of the bangle). This technique is very simple and cheap, but of little accuracy because the bangle assesses the *maximum* arm circumference and not the circumference *halfway* between shoulder and elbow.   It may be useful, however, when resources do not permit any other measurement to be made.

Calculating and tabulating the percentage of the reference value

The reference or "standard" values are shown in Annex 3 (weight-for-height) and Annex 4 (arm-circumference-height).   To calculate the nutritional status of a child, compare the child's weight (or arm circumference) with the values given opposite his height in the relevant table.

This gives the percentage "rank" to which the child belongs, e.g., 70–80%.   For most purposes it is not necessary to know the exact "percentage of reference" for each individual.   Results are most conveniently recorded as shown in Fig. 9.   They can readily be converted into percentages in accordance with the table in the lower right-hand corner of the figure.

Fig. 9 gives a "nutritional profile" indicating the distribution of nutritional status within the population measured.   Without "normal" baseline figures it is not possible to say (unless the situation is extremely good or bad) whether or not a given set of findings is unusual for that population. Results can only be interpreted in this way, if much more information is available, e.g., crop statistics, mortality rates, etc.

The use of local standards of reference is not recommended unless these are based on well-nourished samples *in the same population* prior to the emergency.   *Local standards do not permit international comparisons of value to relief organizations.*

The classification of malnutrition

Body measurements give reasonably accurate estimates of body wasting.   Children below 70% of the reference standard (weight-for-height) can be said with some certainty to be severely malnourished, while those between 70% and 80% are moderately malnourished.

Table 3 shows two classifications using different cut-off points.   In practice, the number and level of the cut-off points will have to be decided arbitrarily, taking two factors into account:

(1) The purpose of the measurement.   If the object is to distinguish children with severe and moderate PEM from normal children for different types of feeding, two cut-off points will be needed.   If a survey is contemplated, divisions by 10% of the reference standard might be used.

(2) The availability of food.   In this case, the cut-off points may be decided (on the basis of a pilot survey) in such a way that the children are classified into groups according to the food available to feed them.

Different techniques give different rates of malnutrition. For instance, if a cut-off point of 80% arm-circumference-for-height is used, this will often give a higher "rate" for malnutrition than will 80% weight-for-height. (In many countries where chronic malnutrition is common, 90%, 80%, 70% weight-for-height are very roughly equivalent to 80%, 70%, 60% weight-for-age respectively.)

TABLE 3. EXAMPLES OF CLASSIFICATION

	Arm circumference (AC) [a] (cm)	AC-for-height (% of reference standard)	Weight-for-height [b] (% of reference standard)
A. Three categories			
Well nourished and mild PEM	13.5 or more	85% or more	80% or more
Moderate PEM	12.5–13.5	70–85%	70–80%
Severe PEM	under 12.5	under 70%	under 70%
B. Two categories			
Well nourished and mild PEM	13 or more	75% or more	80% or more
Clearly malnourished	less than 13	under 75%	less than 80%

[a] Arm circumference might be used alone for children under 5, although this is not recommended. A child would be classified as malnourished if the AC was less than a minimum acceptable value (cut-off point).
[b] Cut-off points 2 or 3 standard deviations below the reference median have recently been recommended (see Annex 3).

Organization of individual screening

Objectives

First decide what criteria (e.g., weight-for-height, arm-circumference-for-height, QUAC stick measurements, oedema) are to be used for the screening. When body measurements are used and the choice is between four courses of action (e.g., no assistance, weekly ration, daily ration, and intensive supervised feeding), four categories of classification should be established.

There is, for instance, very little point in selecting a large number of malnourished children unless facilities are available and organized for them. Obtain a rough estimate of the proportion of malnourished children in a large population by quickly measuring 200 children (see Annex 6).

Decide which population is to be screened. This will depend upon the local situation, but remember that people attending relief centres are not necessarily the worst off. Malnourished individuals may remain at home, because they are unable to walk, live in relatively inaccessible areas, or, in the case of marasmic children, are not regarded by their parents as being in need of help.

Procedure

Inform the community through local leaders at least 24 hours in advance to allow them to arrange for all eligible people to attend. Choose a time that is convenient for the community.

When large numbers of people are to be screened, make sure that they are well organized and, if at all possible, sitting down out of the sun. Convert existing buildings, wherever possible, into temporary screening locations.

Select the severely malnourished first, by clinical examination. If people are well organized, this can be done very quickly by walking along rows. Do not keep severely ill people waiting for long periods of time.

Use a system of individual identification, i.e., date-stamp the feeding card or mark the individual's finger nail with a 10% silver nitrate solution.

Use clearly defined criteria for selection, e.g., pregnant and lactating women, the very old, and/or all children shorter than some designated height—105 cm is the approximate average height of a 5-year-old.

Make sure each individual understands what is being done. Food may be distributed immediately as the direct result of a screening. In this case, the individual should be shown to the appropriate distribution point.

Screening may be done on each occasion that food is distributed or intermittently, in which case each individual (or family) is given a card that entitles him to food at several subsequent distributions.

If whole communities are being screened, *record* the results. These can be useful for making comparisons with future measurements. *Record* the results of other observations, e.g., oedema (Fig. 10).

Staff and equipment

A team of six workers given one day's training can screen from 500 to 2000 persons a day. Efficiency decreases in sparsely populated areas. It is quicker to use the QUAC stick (AC-for-height) than weight-for-height.

The equipment needs for each measuring team are:

2 tape-measures (ideally of fibreglass or locally made), if AC is to be measured

1 scale with an adequate support (table or tripod) and 1 spare

1 measuring stick and a baby-board to measure height (or length)

a known weight to check the accuracy of the scales (e.g., a piece of metal or solid rock)

ration cards, special ration entitlements, etc.

2 rubber date-stamps, one official stamp to validate the ration card (important for preventing abuses), a table, and a chair

tally forms for recording oedema or other signs (Fig. 10) and the number of children falling into different nutritional categories. Lactating or pregnant women should not be classified with females of 10-54 years but in a special category. The tabulation is completed at the end of the day and the percentage of oedema per age group and sex is entered on a special form.

FIG. 10. OEDEMA TALLY FORM

Group	Height (cm)	Male		Female	
		No oedema	Oedema	No oedema	Oedema
Unable to walk (0 −1 years)	under 75	IIII	I	III	I
Preschool children (1−4 years)	75 - 105	ꐃꐃꐃ[a]	IIII	ꐃꐃ II	IIII
School children (5−9 years)	105 - 136	IIII	II	III	II
Active population[b] (10−54 years)	over 136	ꐃꐃ I		ꐃꐃ	
55 years or more		ꐃꐃ III	I	ꐃꐃ ꐃꐃ I	
Lactating women				ꐃꐃ	II
Pregnant women				III	I
TOTAL		27	8	37	10

[a] ꐃꐃ = 5.
[b] Excluding lactating or pregnant women.

WHO 77817

Organization of nutritional surveillance[1]

Under most circumstances the nutritional status of preschool children can be taken to reflect the nutritional status of the whole community. However, adults also suffer from food shortages and in cultures where the feeding of children has precedence over that of the parents, it may be the adults who are most affected by starvation.

Weight-for-height is a suitable measurement for adults between 15 and 50 years old. However, the range of values which can be regarded as normal is much wider for this age group than for young children (see Annex 3).

To measure changes in the nutritional status of a large population accurately over a period of time requires exacting sampling standards and techniques (see Annex 6).

However, some useful information can be obtained by relatively simple methods.

---

[1] The surveillance of communicable diseases is dealt with in Chapter 7.

(a) *Where vulnerable groups are periodically screened for food distribution, using body measurement or other indicators*

Data collected during screenings can be recorded and comparisons made between measurements. Results of anthropometric measurements should be arranged by 10% groupings (see Fig. 9), and converted to percentages. This gives "nutritional profiles" of the community on two or more occasions. These can be compared directly to see if the proportion of the malnourished is changing, and in what way.

If part of the population is being screened *and* having food distributed to it, this group is obviously not representative of the population at large. The required information can only be obtained by sample surveys (see Annex 6).

Comparisons between two measurements taken from the same community should be interpreted with caution. The fact that the death rate for malnourished children is generally very high may lead to a false impression of improvement. For example:

	First measurement	*Second measurement*
Number over 80 % of reference standard	36	1 death . . 35
Number under 80 % of reference standard	12 (25 %)	6 deaths . . 6 (15 %)

Here, there seems to have been an improvement whereas in fact the situation may have deteriorated.

N.B. A real improvement might be caused by climatic or economic factors *in spite* of an inefficient food relief programme.

Even small differences in the procedure used during a screening may cause a different group of people to attend. If the first screening is held early in the morning the group measured will be different from that measured at a second screening held at midday, when people are at work. The differences introduced by such variations can be very large and lead to false conclusions.

Indicators other than body measurements can be used for screening, either singly or in combination. Since organization and travelling take up so much working time, several indicators should be estimated on the same occasion, e.g., oedema, specific signs of vitamin deficiency.

(b) *Where vulnerable groups are not regularly screened*

Data collected weekly at fixed health facilities and maternal and child health centres can give some idea of changes, e.g., number and complaints of individuals attending for health care or nutritional relief. Data of this kind should be used with caution because they do not give a picture of the whole population but only of those who

— feel that they need *medical* attention, whatever the reason

— can physically attend the health facilities (e.g., live within walking distance, etc.).

Local auxiliaries can be temporarily recruited and trained to carry out the surveillance of simple symptoms and signs of malnutrition at the camp or village level.

The training can, for instance, be organized as follows:

1 day: major signs of PEM (wasting, oedema)
        investigation of night blindness
        diagnosis of major eye lesions due to vitamin A deficiency
        clinical signs of other vitamin deficiencies
1 day: drill in measuring weight (or arm circumference) and height reporting
        system
1 day: field test

Visiting schedules for auxiliaries must be carefully prepared by a census of the dwellings (houses, tents) involved. Conclusions based on a poorly organized and supervised surveillance system are not valid.

On completing a regular cycle of visits, the auxiliary will report the total number of families and children visited as well as the number of persons presenting the selected signs, by age and sex. Rates should be calculated centrally.

Other indicators for the evaluation of relief programmes

The following indicators can be useful in evaluating a relief programme:

● Age distribution of children attending relief centres compared with the age distribution from census data.

● Monthly attendance rate of children registered. This is obtained by dividing the monthly average number of those attending by the total number of children registered.

● Malnutrition rates in people attending relief centres compared with similar rates obtained by an occasional survey of random samples and house-to-house visits in the same area. This indicator is essential in confirming that the programme is really reaching the target groups.

The following data can be obtained from analysis of a random sample of registration cards or growth charts:

● Percentage of children losing weight over 1 month. Weight gain over a long period of time is no proof of a successful programme. Undernourished children may gain some weight and still fall into a lower nutritional category.
● Percentage of children shifting to another nutritional category in a given period of time (e.g., from 70–80% weight-for-height up to 80–90% or down to 60–70%). This information can easily be taken from the simplified growth chart (Fig. 11).
● Weight gain processed as weight gain ÷ last weight, the results being expressed as g/kg.

The daily weight gain in "normal" reference children between 1 and 5 years old is about 1 g/kg. In malnourished children, the gain must be higher to indicate recovery.

FIG. 11. SIMPLIFIED GROWTH CHART [a]

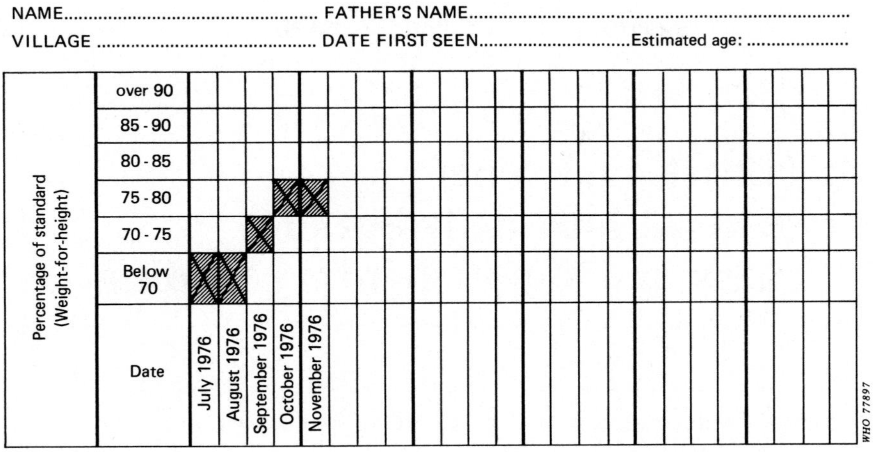

NAME.. FATHER'S NAME...

VILLAGE .... DATE FIRST SEEN.............................Estimated age: ....

Percentage of standard (Weight-for-height)	over 90																							
	85 - 90																							
	80 - 85																							
	75 - 80			▨	▨																			
	70 - 75		▨																					
	Below 70	▨	▨																					
	Date	July 1976	August 1976	September 1976	October 1976	November 1976																		

WHO 77897

[a] Adapted from: CAPONE, C. A growth surveillance system for food and nutrition programs. In: *Integrating Title II program with locally operated nutrition, socio-economic and humanitarian activities*. Catholic Relief Services, 1977 (mimeographed).
This chart is to be used in conjunction with the nutritional status chart (Fig. 9). Kept by the mother, it can be printed on the reverse side of a ration card. The information is recorded weekly or monthly.

4. Nutritional relief: general food distribution, mass and supplementary feeding

There are four ways in which food relief may be organized:

1. *General food distribution.* Dry food is distributed to people who are able to prepare their own meals.

2. *Mass feeding.* Prepared meals from a central kitchen are served to the population.

3. *Supplementary feeding.* In addition to the ration (dry foods or meals) for the whole family, vulnerable groups receive an *extra* meal or ration to meet their particular needs.

4. Intensive or therapeutic feeding of PEM cases (Chapter 5).

Food must be nutritionally valuable as well as acceptable to the local population. Remember that foods that are *not* consumed have no nutritional value!

Average rations must be calculated to provide at least 6.3 MJ (1500 kcal$_{th}$)/person/day for a few weeks and 7.5 MJ (1800 kcal$_{th}$)/person/day for longer periods.

Organization and planning (ration cards, distribution schedule) are the keys to the success or failure of a relief programme.

There are four ways in which food relief may be distributed:

1. general food distribution (dry rations);
2. mass feeding (cooked meals);
3. supplementary feeding of vulnerable groups;
4. therapeutic feeding (see Chapter 5).

The type of food distribution employed will depend entirely upon local circumstances. A refugee camp, where individuals have cooking facilities, may be adequately served by the distribution of dry rations alone, possibly with supplementary food for the vulnerable groups. Where a large rural population is affected but can find a proportion of its food locally, a range of programmes will be needed, e.g., some people with full rations, some with partial rations and selected groups with supplementary rations.

● Wherever possible, assist people at their homes and avoid setting up refugee camps, though the latter step may sometimes be unavoidable (in the case of flood victims, refugees from conflicts, etc.). Camps are very difficult to disperse. Do not create camps just because they are administratively more convenient.

● Distributing food to nomadic groups is difficult, and no easy way of doing so has been found. Points at which people congregate (e.g., water sources) may be selected as the best places at which to distribute food; alternatively, large amounts of food may be given out (100 kg) at each distribution if this avoids setting up refugee camps.

The distribution of centrally prepared meals may be indicated when:

— people do not have basic cooking equipment;
— not enough fuel (e.g., firewood) is available for individual cooking;
— it is necessary to check who is eating the food, as in supervised supplementary feeding.

Providing cooked food on a mass scale requires a high level of organization if the number of people is greater than, say, 2000 or if they are scattered over large areas.

The supplementary feeding of vulnerable groups consists in providing food to supplement the deficiencies in calories and/or nutrients of the basic diet consumed.

Basic considerations in selecting foods

The food must:

(*a*) correspond to the nutritional needs and food habits of the beneficiaries;
(*b*) fulfil special logistic requirements, i.e., be easy to transport, store, and distribute; and
(*c*) be available in sufficient quantities.

General food distribution

Specific requirements in selecting foods

— In addition to the general concepts stressed above, foods should be as few in number as possible.

— Unfamiliar types of food are often given as aid. If these are useful nutritionally but unacceptable to the population, it may help if those in charge arrange a public demonstration at which they explain what the foods are and, in the presence of local leaders, sample them themselves.

— Where a population is entirely dependent upon relief, include items like tea, sugar, and spices as part of the ration. In this case especially, it is essential that food be given against some kind of return from the recipient whenever possible.

Calculating dry rations

This is best done on a *family*—rather than an individual—basis, since in this way the number of people attending distributions will be reduced and administration simplified. Distribution is also made easier if rations are calculated on the following scale rather than based on the exact age distribution of the family: up to 5 members, 5–8 members, 9 or more members, etc.; and/or if two levels of ration are provided—e.g., under 10 years old (or height under 130 cm), 5.4 MJ (1300 kcal$_{th}$); over 10 years old, 8.4 MJ (2000 kcal$_{th}$) (this corresponds to an overall average of 7.5 MJ (1800 kcal$_{th}$) per day per person).

If the amount of relief food available for distribution is insufficient, a lower energy intake may have to be set for the assisted population, for instance, 6.3 MJ (1500 kcal$_{th}$)/person/day, or even less. The ideal or recommended intake of 9.8 MJ (2350 kcal$_{th}$) (Annex 1) is often impossible to achieve in times of acute food shortage. It may also be considered inappropriate to provide this amount to the part of the population assisted by the relief programme, while those who are not eligible for assistance have to make do with their usual very low level of energy intake.

"Reduced ration" can be used when people are able to provide some of the staple food,[1] e.g., cereals, for themselves or in the phasing-out period

---

[1] A staple food is one that is normally consumed in a country or community and from which a substantial portion of the total energy intake is derived, especially among the poorer sectors of the population and in times of food shortage.

of a programme. Note the nutritional composition of the reduced ration: two reduced rations may or may *not* be equal to one full ration. Examples:

	Full ration			Reduced ration		
Cereal	400 g	5.9 MJ (1 400 kcal$_{th}$)	40 g protein	100 g	1.5 MJ (350 kcal$_{th}$)	10 g protein
Oil	50 g	1.8 MJ (440 kcal$_{th}$)	0 g protein	50 g	1.8 MJ (440 kcal$_{th}$)	0 g protein
DSM [a]	30 g	0.5 MJ (110 kcal$_{th}$)	11 g protein	50 g	0.7 MJ (180 kcal$_{th}$)	18 g protein
Total	480 g	8.2 MJ (1 950 kcal$_{th}$)	51 g protein	200 g	4.0 MJ (980 kcal$_{th}$)	28 g protein

[a] Dried skim milk.

Organizing a distribution

The key to running a successful food distribution programme is to be well organized. If rations are to be given out to, say, 5000 people, it is unrealistic to expect them to form a queue quietly and take food from openly exposed sacks—chaos would result.

The participation of the community in the relief programme and in decision-making will help towards an orderly distribution. Holding public meetings and keeping the population informed through administrative and natural leaders is essential. However, responsible posts (storekeeping, administration) must be given to reliable individuals outside the community to rule out personal bias, preferences, or vulnerability to pressure.

People should be lined up for distribution and be called—e.g., four at a time—by the guards (villages) or have to pass check-points (camps). If the ground is dry, they should *be seated* in lines. This will prevent pushing and is much less tiring than standing for hours, perhaps in the sun.

(a) Distribution to villages, refugee camps and to nomads

Always inform people well in advance that a food distribution is to occur on a certain day. *Regular* distribution on a fixed day is best and causes least confusion.

A distribution each week or fortnight is recommended because hungry people have difficulty in economizing their food. Also, displaced persons have limited possibilities for storing supplies. Where long journeys are involved, as in the case of nomads, monthly distribution may be indicated.

A reserve supply of empty bags, tins, etc. should be kept for people who are completely destitute, but as a rule people should bring their own receptacles. Bottles and baskets for cereals are usually easily found by the population.

The recipients should always be aware of the amounts they are entitled to: standard measures for cereals and other items should be cut from oil tins (for example), and the weight checked on the scales, and demonstrated in public—if necessary, several times. This will give people a chance to see that there is no cheating and will be economical from the standpoint of control. *Remember to recheck the measures with each new arrival of grain.*

In villages, relief can be distributed through local authorities—village elders, etc.—at a fenced-off spot away from the market place. Family rations should be given, and the distribution based on village registers or official knowledge about families belonging to the village. A simple list can be used; ration cards are not necessary.

A group of villages may have a central store (for food storage, see Chapter 6). Depending on the distance and the transport facilities, village representatives can come in on set days and fetch the rations. Traditional transport—donkeys, camels, boats—should be used if possible.

In a camp, the distribution area should be located near the store and fenced off. People should be served from several lines simultaneously (as many as necessary), each with a check-point for ration cards (Fig. 12). If the camp has, for example, 10 sectors, take sectors 1 and 2 on Monday, 3 and 4 on Tuesday, and so on.

FIG. 12. PLAN FOR DISTRIBUTION OF DRY FOOD

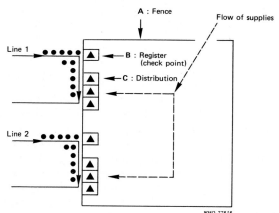

WHO 77818

A. Fence of mats, bamboo, wire, or rope depending on resources and needs. Narrowing aisles for line-ups might also be necessary.
B. Check point for cards. Sheltered by roof (or umbrella). The number of rations is called out clearly to distributors at C.
C. Distribution point. Several bags at a time can be emptied on to a tarpaulin for quicker distribution.

The distribution will be completed in 5 days, allowing 2 days to arrange the store and get new supplies. With a camp twice as big, distribute to sectors 1-5 one week and 6-10 the next. When sudden rains or delayed lorries ruin your plans, inform people *in time*.

FIG. 13. RATION CARD

Example No. 1

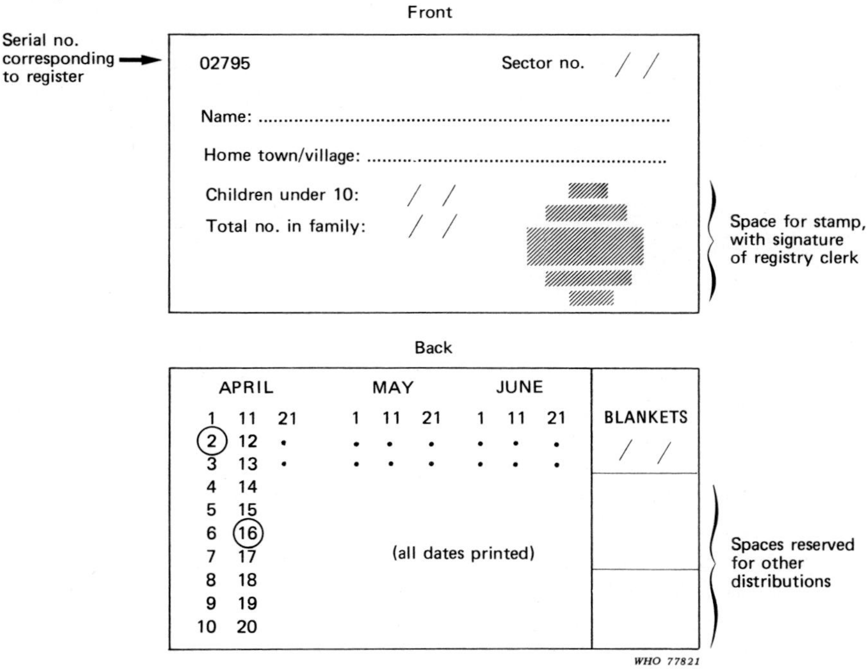

Front

Serial no. corresponding → to register

02795   Sector no. / /

Name: ....

Home town/village: ....

Children under 10:   / /

Total no. in family: / /

) Space for stamp, with signature of registry clerk

Back

APRIL			MAY			JUNE			BLANKETS
1	11	21	1	11	21	1	11	21	
②	12	•	•	•	•	•	•	•	/ /
3	13	•		•	•	•	•	•	
4	14								
5	15								
6	⑯		(all dates printed)						
7	17								
8	18								
9	19								
10	20								

) Spaces reserved for other distributions

WHO 77821

N.B. If another item such as, for instance, soap is issued regularly on this card, the relevant dates can be *crossed out*, as well as or instead of being circled in.

Example No. 2 (adapted from Haitian Red Cross Society ration card).

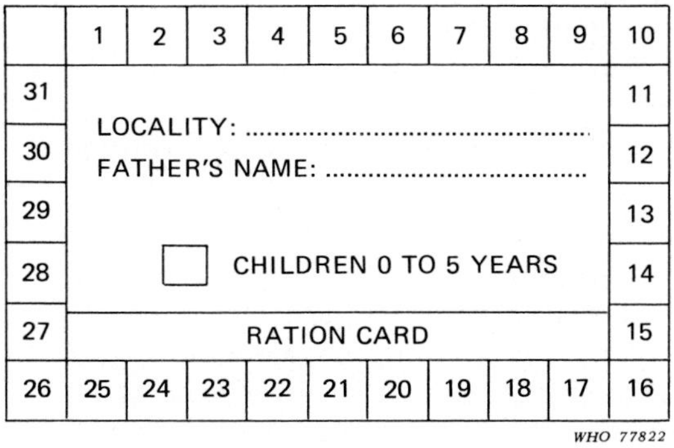

	1	2	3	4	5	6	7	8	9	10
31										11
30	LOCALITY:									12
	FATHER'S NAME:									
29										13
28	☐ CHILDREN 0 TO 5 YEARS									14
27	RATION CARD									15
26	25	24	23	22	21	20	19	18	17	16

WHO 77822

Nomads may be served near the waterholes where they take their animals. Information must be spread early to give them time to come in on the appointed day. An average food ration for each family, or a certain number of bags of cereals, etc. can be issued for distribution within the group, if the nomads are well organized, with accepted leaders.

(b) Identifying individuals—ration cards

To ensure that each individual receives only one ration, some form of identification must be used. In small communities this can be done from names, village lists, etc. With larger numbers of people ration cards must be given out. To ensure that each family receives only one card, distribute these on a house-to-house basis, or at a single distribution attended by the entire population.

A typical ration card is shown in Fig. 13. It should include:
— sector number
— name of head of family and home town/village
— total number of family members
— number of children under 5 (or other suitable age limit)
and on the back, a system for marking rations received, blankets, etc. (Fig. 13, Example 1).

Exchange these cards for new ones every third month: There will always be people who pretend they have "lost" their card, but even if it is a rule never to give a new one, some cases may be found to be genuine and new cards given.

Recording beneficiaries' names and addresses in registers is often time-consuming and ineffective in preventing abuses of the system by the feeding-centre personnel. A simpler system is to use a feeding card with a counterfoil that can be torn off when the ration is received. The number of rations distributed (number of counterfoils) should be compared with the amount of the food actually taken from the store.

Responsibility for the issue of ration cards should be in the hands of a single person. This will save other staff from being bothered when the person in charge is not available.

All ration cards should be marked with a stamp that cannot be forged and is kept by the supervisor. Casual checks should be made at the village market to ascertain whether rations are being sold there.

(c) Food supplies

Order supplies in time.

The following quantities are required for *1000 people*, based on the the examples above). The amounts are given in tonnes (t)—1 t = 1000 kg.

Full ration: 15 t per month per 1000 persons
Reduced ration: 6.3 t per month per 1000 persons.

(d) Staffing and equipment

For each distribution line (see Fig. 12):

1 clerk, 1 person to distribute each food item, at least 2 crowd controllers; ration cards, rubber stamps, receptacles (half petrol-drums, tarpaulins, etc.) for food, standard measures (tins and cans), tables and benches.

Mass feeding (cooked meals)

Mass feeding is usually limited to institutions and refugee camps.

Choice of food

As for dry food distribution.

Every effort should be made to give the normal local diet and, wherever possible, prepare it from foods obtained locally.

The diet should be composed of a staple food (cereal or root), oil or fat (20–40%), legumes and/or animal proteins (DSM), and some vegetables or fruits.

Under ideal circumstances, of each 10 MJ of food served:

— 2–4 MJ should come from fats/oils

— 1 MJ should come from proteins.

If nontraditional food items have to be used, they should be prepared and served in a form as close as possible to local foods (gruel, soup, tortillas, chapatis, etc.).

Spices can increase the acceptability of the food. They are usually cheap and easily available. Use spices in the local fashion whenever possible.

If meat is available, serve it occasionally (e.g., on feast days): this is good for morale.

Calculating food rations

As for the dry food distribution, the *average* daily ration can be between 6.3 MJ or 1500 $kcal_{th}$, (energy minimum, Table 1) and 9.5 MJ or 2350 $kcal_{th}$ (recommended or ideal energy intake, Annex 1).

The quantity to be served is first calculated in terms of dry food (see food composition table in Annex 2) and then in terms of servings (meals). If three meals are served, the total amount of food would normally be broken up in proportions of about 1:2:2 for each meal. For example, if 8.4 MJ (2000 $kcal_{th}$) are given to each individual each day, then 1.7 MJ (400 $kcal_{th}$) would be served for breakfast and 3.3 MJ (800 $kcal_{th}$) for each of the other two meals.

If different servings are prepared for adults and children under 10 years, calculate the amounts of raw food on the basis of 6.3 MJ (1500 kcal$_{th}$) for those under 10 years and 9.2 MJ (2200 kcal$_{th}$) for those over 10 years (overall average = 7.5 MJ (1800 kcal$_{th}$). Children need three meals a day, while two may be sufficient for adults.

If people are able to provide and prepare some food for themselves, reduce the number of daily meals for adults (e.g., one service per day).

Organization of cooking facilities

First, a few questions have to be answered:

1. How many meals are to be prepared at a time?

2. How long in advance can each type of food be prepared?

3. Can the staple food be prepared in a single large batch (e.g., boiled rice), or does it have to be prepared in individual form (e.g., chapatis, tortillas, bread, etc.)?

(a) Kitchens

Kitchens should be set up inside buildings wherever possible. It is often possible to construct a suitable shelter cheaply in the form of either a "lean-to" against some other building or consisting of a roof of thatch or corrugated iron supported on uprights. Except where kitchens are very small, the area should be fenced off to prevent access by the general public. It is always advisable to have as much space as possible for water storage, the washing and cleaning of food, any initial preparation that is required, cooking, the short-term storage of prepared food, and washing up. In a large camp, one kitchen should be set up for each 200–300 families or 1000–1500 people.

(b) Personnel and equipment

Personnel should include cooks (the number would depend on the type and amount of food), cooks' assistants (for cleaning vegetables, making fires, carrying water, etc.), cleaners, and people to wash up. Employ residents of the camps as much as possible (see camp administration, Chapter 8).

Methods of cooking a given staple food usually vary according to the country and even within countries. Local methods and suitable equipment should be employed.

Clearly, foods that can be cooked in bulk will require large receptacles; where large amounts of staple foods have to be baked or fried in individual portions, a larger number of smaller utensils and more personnel will be required.

1. When the food is to be prepared in individual portions, it is necessary first to determine how long each one takes to prepare.   This can be done by timing the preparation of, say, 10 portions by a local cook and then calculating from this the number of cooks, utensils, and cooking points required as follows:

number of portions required for three meals	$= 1000 \times 3 = 3000$
number cooked by one cook in one hour	$= 100$
number of cook hours required	$= 30$
time available for preparation	$= 6$ h
number of cooks required	$= 5 + 2$ (for rest periods) $= 7$

2. When a food is prepared in bulk, calculate as in the following example:

individual (dry) quantity of food	$= 100$ g per meal
maximum volume when cooked	$= 250$ ml
number of people to be fed at one meal	$= 1000$
assuming that the food must be freshly prepared for each meal, then total volume to be prepared twice daily	$= 250$ l

This in practice means that at least two cooking pots about the size of a cut-down petrol drum (200 l) (Fig. 14) and two cooks would be required.

Additional utensils are required for:

— Cooking soup (calculate in the same way as for staple food in bulk)
— mixing, serving, or cleaning ingredients prior to cooking
— fermentation (for example, injera, yoghurt, curd) where this is required
— mixing and serving implements.

At the outset, make a rough calculation of the other utensils required and add to these as experience is gained.

(c) Fires and fuel

If local fuels are being used, e.g., wood or cow dung, then the local system of fire-making is usually the best and should be adopted. If firewood is difficult to obtain, each person or family should be asked to bring one piece to each meal.

(d) Hygiene and food storage

The kitchen and its surroundings must be kept clean. Adequate facilities for the disposal of waste must be provided. It is usually best to employ one or more full-time cleaners and to make them personally responsible for this.

Avoid storing cooked food for any length of time, particularly if the food involved contains meat or other animal products. Some types of local staple foods can be kept safely in an edible condition for several days. Cold-mixed foods, e.g., dried skim milk, should always be made up freshly before use, ideally with boiled cooled water and should never be kept standing or in an uncovered container for more than a few minutes.

Organization of meal distribution

(a) Distribution of cooked meals to families

The registration of families who are to receive cooked rations is similar to the registration procedure for dry ration distribution.

A representative of each family presents a card indicating the number of people to be fed in the family. The ration for the family is measured into a suitable container and the card marked to indicate that the ration has been allocated. It should be remembered that the ration of grain per person will increase in both weight and volume after boiling and the ration should be adjusted accordingly.

In a large community or camp where there are several kitchens and distribution centres, it is important for recipients to know which kitchen they are to attend for feeding. The feeding supervisor should keep a register of all those to be fed from his kitchen. Should a control be necessary, the information in the register should correspond to that on the family feeding card. The card should be marked or, preferably, stamped with the kitchen number. Kitchens should have the number clearly displayed.

FIG. 14. HOW TO USE AN OIL DRUM AS A COOKING UTENSIL

Oil drum (200 litres)   Cooking pot (130 litres)

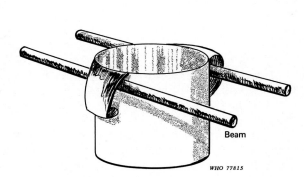

Beam

WHO 77815

(a) Cut the drum following the dotted line, and bend the two sides outwards to permit easy transport with two strong pieces of wood or metal.
(b) Alternatively, cut the drum in half to form two 100-l cooking pots.

(b) Distribution of cooked meals to individuals

Food distributed to individuals should be eaten in an enclosed area under supervision. This is to ensure that all members of the family (particularly the children) eat an adequate ration. This procedure is only praticable in smaller shelters or communities where no more than a few hundred people are to be fed.

A large enclosed area should be constructed, where all the people can assemble at set times each day; alternatively a school-hall or some other suitable building could be used.

If the entire population of the camp or community is to be fed in an enclosed area, no registration card system should be necessary, although those attending should be counted each day.

Only where selective feeding is to be carried out should cards be issued to those in need of feeding.

At well-controlled institutions or camps, plates might be given to each person individually. Either arrange for these to be washed centrally or provide facilities for each person to wash his own.

Supplementary feeding

The purpose of supplementary feeding is to supplement deficiencies in energy and/or nutrients, especially protein, in the basic diet of those more vulnerable to malnutrition: children under 5, pregnant or lactating women, medical cases, old people, children selected by a screening method.

Supplementary feeding can take two forms:

— distribution of a dry ration to vulnerable groups in addition to the general ration given to the whole family ("carry-home" system)

— "On-the-spot" feeding of an additional meal to ensure that the right food reaches only the selected group.

Choice of foods and beneficiaries

Foods are selected for their particular nutritional value. An appropriate ration is, for example:

- 40 g dry skim milk (0.7 MJ or 160 $kcal_{th}$) plus
  50 g cereal-based special food (Chapter 6) or rolled oats (0.8 MJ or 200 $kcal_{th}$)
  or
- 100 g rolled oats or cereal based special food (1.7 MJ or 400 $kcal_{th}$)
  or
- 40 g dry skim milk plus 20 g oil (total: 1.4 MJ or 340 $kcal_{th}$).

As a guideline: around 1.5 MJ (350 $kcal_{th}$) and 15 g protein constitute a usual supplement in relief programme.

Vulnerable groups are the target of any supplementary programme. While all children under 5 years old are vulnerable, special attention should be given to the age group 0–2 years.

Breast-feeding. Mothers need sufficient food to maintain or resume their milk production. If the child cannot get its mother's milk, a substitute should be sought. Any woman who has recently breast-fed can reinstitute her milk production simply by letting the infant suck at her breast very frequently (approximately 10 times a day, some minutes at each side every time) for several days. If a "substitute mother" is not found, artificial feeding should be given, preferably by cup and spoon. *Bottle-feeding must be reserved for exceptional cases* (e.g., where there is a very young child and complete failure of lactation) and be administered under the close supervision of relief personnel. Under *no* circumstances must artificial feeds be prepared in advance and left at room temperature.

From the fourth to sixth month onwards, the infant needs some foods *in addition to the mother's milk.*

Supplementary feeding must be given both to lactating mothers (for milk production) and to children above 4 months of age (to meet their increasing requirements).

Organization of a "carry-home" system

This is similar to a general ration distribution. The education of the mothers and the regular measurement of the nutritional status of the children will increase children's chances of receiving the food meant for them. Whenever possible (e.g., in camps), mothers should bring along all their children when fetching supplementary rations so that they can be examined. Almost inevitably there will be some sharing within the family, so that it might be necessary to increase the ration.

Organization of "on-the-spot" feeding

Here, vulnerable groups attend regularly (usually daily) to receive a meal (perhaps a simple supplement of, say, DSM) which must be eaten on the spot and not carried home. The supplementary meal is given in *addition* to the normal meals given in the family. Inform the parents so that the children still get their normal share of family meals.

Choose a time for food distribution that does not coincide with normal family mealtimes.

The object of on-the-spot feeding is to ensure that particular individuals receive the food and that it is not subdivided within the family.

Individual ration cards

In a "carry-home" system, ration cards are necessary (see Fig. 13 and 15).

In a programme of supplementary meals for *all* children in a camp, cards should be avoided as they damage easily. Instead, each child could get a number marked on a piece of metal, cloth, or other resistant material, the numbers being crossed off a stencilled list (or blackboard) during the distribution. Feeding points should be within walking distance for small children and the individual numbers referred to each point by different colours or other symbols. No register is necessary if all children under a certain age (or height) are included.

FIG. 15. SUPPLEMENTARY FEEDING CARD [a]

| NAME .... No. .... SECTOR ☐ |
| AGE............................ SEX ☐F ☐M |
| FATHER'S NAME .... |
| MOTHER'S NAME .... |

APRIL	MAY	JUNE
1 11 21 2 12 22 3 13 23 4 14 24 5 15 25 6 16 26 7 17 27 8 18 28 9 19 29 10 20 30		

WHO 77823

[a] For reverse side, see Fig. 11 (simplified growth chart) or indicate: date, weight, height, % weight-for-height, remarks (treatment, dry food supplement, etc.).

In supplementary feeding programmes for selected groups of children, the point of checking is not to prevent children from being served twice, but to ascertain their regular attendance at meals.

These children should have individual cards and be listed in a register by camp sector, so that helpers can easily find them if they fail to show up. As children in this category are normally taken to meals by their mothers or elder sisters or brothers, their cards should suffer less in handling. It is useful to have a combined card for feeding and follow-up (Fig. 15).

5. Therapeutic feeding

PEM is treated by giving food of high nutritional value. Give 0.6–0.8 MJ (150–200 $kcal_{th}$) and 2–3 g of protein per kg body weight. Reduced feeding is recommended for the first few days.

For the first few days, close supervision and feedings every three hours on a 24-hour basis are necessary. Mothers should cooperate and feed their sick children themselves.

Medical treatment and drug administration must be limited to essential items.

Infection and dehydration are the major causes of death, which often occurs within the first four days. Antibiotic treatment of infections and close supervision are essential. Immunization against measles is recommended.

Criteria of recovery are:

oedema loss, weight gain and improvement of general condition.

Failure is mainly due to faulty feeding or to infection.

This chapter presents the *basic concepts of therapeutic feeding* in severe cases of protein-energy malnutrition (PEM). Therapeutic feeding is required to reduce deaths among infants and young children with severe PEM.

Criteria for admission

- Severe marasmus or oedema (kwashiorkor), or
- Weight-for-height less than 70% of the reference (or AC-for-height less than 75%, or arm circumference (AC) less than 12 cm).

When facilities are very limited, the weight-for-height standard may be lowered to 65% or even to 60% and uncomplicated cases can be treated at home, if seen daily.

Day-care centres; residential centres

There are two types of therapeutic feeding, depending on the setting.

At residential centres: feeding on a 24-hour basis (inpatient). Mothers must be admitted, that is, accommodated and fed with children suffering from severe malnutrition and, *if necessary*, they should be allowed to bring along other children.

At day-care centres: four meals a day on an ambulatory (outpatient) basis.

Severe cases of PEM can be admitted to an improvised centre, where results are better and cost is lower than in non-specialized hospitals. Intensive feeding *day and night* is essential in the first stage of treatment.

Lay-out of a residential feeding centre (30 children)

Local material (e.g., mud, wooden huts, tents, etc.) or existing buildings (schools, etc.) should be used. Accommodation should, if possible, conform to traditional local standards. Fig. 16 shows a residential therapeutic feeding centre with a day-care section. The actual layout can be simplified if local circumstances require it. In practice, any large building or facility can be converted into a feeding centre.

FIG. 16. RESIDENTIAL FEEDING CENTRE WITH DAY-CARE SECTION

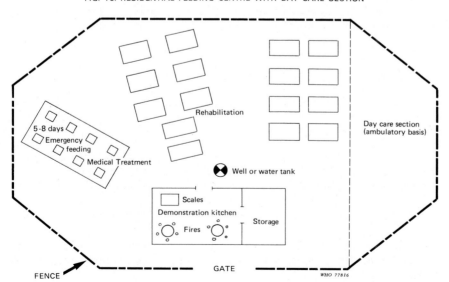

Emergency section (8–10 children)

The children (and mothers) are accommodated in one single large hut or ward (class-room). Close supervision by qualified personnel—nurses, for instance—is required on a full-time basis.

As soon as a child no longer requires constant supervision, he is transferred to the section "rehabilitation with special attention" (5–8 days after admission).

Rehabilitation (20–25 children)

Separate local accommodation is provided for the children and accompanying relatives. Feeding is provided *by the mothers* under the supervision of auxiliaries. Qualified supervision is required on a periodic basis (detection and prevention of complications). Local foods in semiliquid form are introduced, and the frequency of feedings decreased (4–6 meals a day).

Therapeutic feeding

The child must be weighed on admission, daily for one week, and every week thereafter.

During the first week, the child cannot assimilate a full ration; it is recommended to give 0.4 MJ (100 kcal$_{th}$) and 2 g of high-quality protein per kg of body weight divided into 8 meals (every 3 hours). As soon as the child's general condition permits (generally after 5–7 days), 0.6–0.8 MJ (150–200 kcal$_{th}$) and about 3 g protein (depending on the quality) are required per kg of body weight to achieve the most rapid rate of recovery. When a patient does not tolerate an increase in the size of the portion, it is best to return to a more dilute formula and/or reduce the volume.

On admission	On discharge
3-hourly feeling (day and night) ⟶	3–5 meals/day
liquid food ⟶	semi-solid
special diets ⟶	local foods enriched with skim milk or CSM

While increased energy intake will speed up recovery, there is little benefit in increasing the intake of protein above the levels indicated.

Standard preparations should contain approximately 4.2 MJ/l (1 kcal$_{th}$/ml), and 20–25 ml per kg of weight should be given at each meal. Any preparation of high nutritional value can be used for the treatment of PEM.

In severe cases, the patient should be fed on a high-protein and high-energy liquid diet every three hours (day and night) in the first week of treatment.

Suitable preparations

Milk-based diet. To prepare, carefully mix together 80 g of dried skim milk (DSM), 40 g sugar, and 50 g edible oil. Boiled cooled water is added slowly to make one litre; stir constantly. The mixture contains about 30 g protein and 3.7 MJ (900 kcal$_{th}$) per litre. This type of preparation is readily available.

K Mix II. This is a standard UNICEF formula made of calcium caseinate 17 g, DSM 28 g, and sugar 55 g, with the required daily allowance of vitamin A. It has the advantage of a low lactose content but is poor in iron and some vitamins. First, 100 g of K Mix II and 60 g edible oil are mixed well together (the oil is absolutely essential). Boiled warm water is added to make one litre. Stir well. The mixture contains about 30 g protein and about 3.7 MJ (900 kcal$_{th}$) per litre. K Mix II should *only* be used *to initiate the treatment* as it is very expensive.

In general:

Any food preparation can be used if containing no less than 20 g good-quality protein and 3.7 MJ (900 kcal$_{th}$)/l; 20–40 % of the calorie intake should be provided by oil.

Sugar can be partly replaced by thoroughly cooked, dried, and finely pounded cereals.

Oil provides "compact" calories (37.6 MJ/kg or 9 kcal$_{th}$/g). Between 40 and 60 g can be used for one litre of liquid food. Red palm oil is rich in provitamin A but does not mix well.

Depending on the local climate and the quality of the oil, a *dry* mixture (oil included) can be prepared several days in advance.

Liquid preparations must not be kept for more than 6 hours.

Administration of food

The feeding of sick children demands great patience.

● Use a cup and/or spoon (avoid bottle-feeding in tropical countries).

● After 3–5 days, semi-solid food can be given instead of liquid food. A milk-based diet or special foods (Chapter 6) should progressively replace K Mix II, which is not a complete food and should be reserved for the initial treatment of PEM.

● Feeding should be attempted even in the presence of occasional vomiting.

● A nasogastric tube can be used for up to 4 days. Indications are: no appetite, vomiting, lack of cooperation by the mother, failure to gain weight. However, it is an emergency measure which should not be used unless really necessary.

A moistened tube (internal diameter 2 mm, length 50 cm) is introduced by a nurse into the nose and fed down the throat and into the stomach.   The passage of the tube into the oesophagus is easiest if the patient swallows.   It is essential to check that the tube is in the stomach and not in the lungs.   This can be done by removing a small amount of clear fluid from the tube by a syringe.   Alternatively, inject a few cm^3 of air into the tube; if the tube is in the stomach, a loud bubbling noise will be heard in the child's abdomen.   The tube should be secured to the temple or cheek with sticking plaster.   After carefully checking that the tube is in the stomach, the normal volume of liquid food can be fed slowly down the tube by means of a large syringe (50 cm^3).   After the feed, the tube is rinsed through with a few cm^3 of clean water and can then be left or else removed and replaced at the next feed.   Oral medicines can also be given through a nasogastric tube.

Medical care and medicines

> Food is the specific drug against PEM

Medical care is dealt with more fully in Chapter 7.

The following points may be helpful to those responsible for therapeutic feeding centres.

● No drugs should be given unless they are absolutely essential. Observation has shown that staff may waste considerable time in giving inessential and expensive medicines instead of supervising intensive feeding.

● Treatment by antibiotics must be limited to treatment of identified infections. Infection is often masked in malnourished children, and hypothermia rather than fever may be present. Procaine penicillin is the first drug of choice.

● Anthelmintics can be administered routinely after 5–7 days of emergency feeding.

● A measles outbreak in a feeding centre can be disastrous. The immunization of patients with severe PEM against measles is a priority as soon as their condition has started to improve.

● Administration of a high dose of vitamin A (see Chapter 2) should be a routine procedure if dietary vitamin A deficiency is suspected in the area.

● The daily administration of iron with folic acid (UNICEF tablets) is recommended.

● Multivitamin preparations can be of some assistance. It is, however, preferable to prevent, or give specific treatment for, the mineral or vitamin deficiencies prevalent in the area.

● If available, potassium chloride should be added to each feeding, especially in the case of diarrhoea (which is frequent during the first days). A bulk solution can be prepared with 7.5 g in 100 ml of water; 5 ml/kg of body weight are given daily in divided doses.

Signs of recovery and criterion for discharge

Oedema loss (kwashiorkor). Usually after 5–10 days. Oedema loss is accompanied by a loss of weight due to elimination of water.

Weight gain. Children with PEM (kwashiorkor patients after the oedema loss) should show *a weight gain of 8–10 g per kg every day.* (The standard weight gain for a normal 1-year-old child is 1 g per kg per day.)

Improvement in general condition. Increasing appetite, alert behaviour, normal stools. Progress must be assessed daily if possible or at least every 2–3 days. Weights should be measured at least each week and recorded on a chart for each child; mothers should be given a careful explanation of the meaning of the chart. The patient can be discharged when he reaches 90% of the weight of a reference child of the same *height* (90% weight-for-height).

Complications

Death occurs in 10–20% of cases and usually takes place within the first 4 days. Infection and dehydration are the major causes.

Other possible complications are:

— Failure to gain weight

— Hypothermia (the temperature of the body is lower than normal—i.e., under 36°C)

— Severe anaemia

— Lactose intolerance (intolerance to the sugar of non-human milks)

— Hypoglycaemia (lack of sugar in the blood)

— Relapses.

Failure to gain weight

With high-energy feeding, most malnourished children recover after 4–5 weeks, i.e., they reach 90% or more of the reference weight for their height. Sometimes children fail to respond to treatment and do not gain weight satisfactorily. Here there are two possibilities: (1) there is some problem with the actual feeds (generally they are not prepared properly or else they are inadequate in quantity or frequency); (2) there is a medical problem (e.g., an infection, worm infestation, tuberculosis, etc.). Medical examination and/or nasogastric feeding are indicated if there is no oedema loss or weight gain after one week. In areas where tuberculosis is common, any malnourished child who does not gain weight satisfactorily despite a good dietary intake should be suspected of and treated for tuberculosis.

Hypothermia

Malnourished children, particularly marasmic ones, tend to have a low body temperature, especially at night. Care should be taken to ensure that the children are warm at night, even though the air temperature may seem uncomfortably high to the staff. Mothers should be encouraged to hold their children close to their bodies at night.

Severe anaemia

Anaemia is often severe and can deteriorate even after treatment for PEM has been given for 1 or 2 weeks. In severe cases, blood transfusion is recommended. Routine administration of iron with folic acid is recommended for the duration of the stay in the centre to prevent acute deterioration (ferrous sulfate solution or tablets: 150 mg + 100 μg of folic acid per day in two doses).

Lactose intolerance

Profuse diarrhoea can, in some regions, be attributed to a lower tolerance to cow's milk sugar (lactose). Most diarrhoeas, however, are caused not by lactose intolerance but by infection. If lactose intolerance is suspected, confirmation should be obtained by withholding milk from the feeds; should the condition be present, diarrhoea will stop within 12 hours and start again after milk is reintroduced.

If lactose intolerance is confirmed, a low-lactose diet can be given (K Mix II, sour milk, yoghurt, nonmilk diets). If lactose intolerance is not confirmed, there is no contraindication to giving the milk-based diet as recommended, or two-hourly feedings of 20 ml/kg of half-strength milk-based diet for a few days.

Hypoglycaemia (low blood glucose)

This is less common when feedings are given at regular intervals during the night. Oral (or, if necessary, intravenous) administration of a strong sugar (glucose, dextrose, or sucrose) solution will be effective almost immediately. This *must* be followed by frequent oral feeds of sugar, or relapse may occur.

Relapses

Relapses after discharge from the feeding centre are very frequent (up to 75% of cases) unless the mother is admitted with the child and has taken over the feeding of the child herself. Failure to educate the mother can make intensive feeding meaningless.

Hygiene

Children suffering from PEM are very vulnerable to all infections.

● Safe boiled water should be available in large quantities (at least 20 litres per person). Clean cooking utensils, measures, and containers with warm antiseptic (chlorine) or detergent solution should also be available.

● Do not reconstitute feeds in advance. Protect them from flies, insects, and dust.

● Mothers should clean the child's feeding plate and utensils every day.

● Hand-washing with soap is essential before feeding the child.

● Latrine facilities should be provided for patients and staff.

Facilities and equipment

These should be as simple and inexpensive as possible (use local material).

Facilities should be isolated by a fence (e.g., bamboo, tarpaulin); there should be one or two wards (total 40 m²) for emergency feeding, individual traditional shelters measuring 2 × 12 m (for child, mother, and other children if necessary). Water (well or large tank), one demonstration kitchen (30 m² with traditional stoves and fuel) plus one storage room (15 m² with a lock), and latrines for the staff and patients. Accommodation and eating place for staff, if necessary.

Equipment needs for 30 children are:

— 35 beds. Young children can sleep with the mother unless on a drip or nasogastric feeding. Tarpaulins and mats for the floor are useful.

— Blankets, safe places for the mothers' belongings.

— 25 lanterns (with fuel) for staff and mothers (night-feeding).

— 5 pots (with covers), 1 griddle, stoves and fuel (to prepare food for emergency feeding six times a day).

— 5 buckets, 5 stirrers, 5 measuring-cups.

— 100 feeding-cups and spoons (mothers should be encouraged to bring their own utensils).

— 25 nasogastric tubes with adhesive tape, 25 plastic syringes (50 cm³) for feeding (if glass syringes are used, more will be needed).

— 2 accurate beam-balances (one in the emergency section, one in the demonstration kitchen) plus one spare, an adequate supply of growth charts, forms, pencils, pens, paper, measuring sticks, and baby-boards.
— Minimum standardized medical equipment and drugs for *paediatric* use (see Chapter 7).

Staffing

For the recommended number of about 30 resident children, reasonable staffing is required to maintain day-and-night emergency feeding:

— 1 experienced nurse (or medical student) full-time
— 1 nursing aid (for the emergency ward)
— 2 health workers to train mothers and supervise feeding
— labourers or helpers.

A medical officer can visit up to 10 centres (for overall supervision, as well as medical examination of problem cases) if travelling distances are small. Personnel should be recruited from the population affected. Labourers should be trained to perform specific, well-defined tasks. Accommodation must be provided for night-duty personnel. Feeding and handling of the children must be left to the mothers.

6. Special foods

Relief workers are often sent unfamiliar processed foods. Special foods are convenient but should supplement, not replace, the local diet.

In general, 100 g of special food provides approximately 1.5 MJ (360 kcal$_{th}$) and 20 g of protein. Vitamins are often added.

The most common of the special foods are the dried milks (skimmed, that is, with no vitamins A–D, unless fortified, or full-cream with vitamins A–D), the blends such as Corn–Soy Milk (CSM) and Wheat-Soy Blend (WSB), and the parboiled cereals (bulgur wheat).

Inappropriate foods must be returned or destroyed.

During emergencies, relief workers are often sent unfamiliar processed foods.

Foods prepared locally with local ingredients are preferable to imported special foods and are best adapted to the specific cultural conditions.[1]

Most special foods are intended for vulnerable groups as supplements to the local diet. They should not replace the traditional diet but supplement it. Processed foods are very convenient to distribute and prepare.

Special imported foods should be replaced as soon as possible by locally grown and prepared supplements of the same nutritional value.

Blended foods may not be familiar to the population. Prepare a demonstration in which all the ingredients are displayed separately. When given without an explanation or a demonstration of how to cook them, they may be thrown away.

---

[1] For recipes, see: CAMERON, M. & HOFVANDER, Y. *Manual on feeding infants and young children.* 2nd edition. New York, Protein-Calorie Advisory Group of the United Nations System, 1976.

TABLE 4. SPECIAL PROCESSED FOODS

Type of food	Average nutritional values [a] per 100 g		Minimum cooking time (min) after adding to boiling water	Remarks
	MJ/kcal_th	Protein (g)		
Blends of cereals, legumes, and dry skim milk				
CSM (Corn-Soy Milk)	1.6/370	20	5–10	CSM and WSM are supplied in
Instant CSM	1.6/380	20	Instant CSM is fully pre-cooked (ready to mix)	22.5-kg multiwall paper bags (the outer wall is impregnated with insecticides and moderately resistant to moisture); dimensions 51 × 84 × 25.5 cm.
WSM (Wheat-Soy Milk)	1.5/360	20	5–10	
Superamine (Algeria only)	1.4/340	20	5–10	Vitamins and minerals added (except in the case of Faffa).
Faffa (Ethiopia only)	1.4/340	20	5–10	
Blends of cereals and legumes				
WSB (Wheat-Soy Blend)	1.5/360	20	5–10	These foods do not contain cow's milk.
SF bul (Soy-Fortified bulgur)	1.5/350	17	20 less, if soak-ed over night	Vitamins and minerals added to WSB, SFCM, incaparina, balahar, and SWF.
SFCM (Soy-Fortified Corn Meal)	1.6/390	13	15	SF bul is not a flour (cracked grains of bulgur wheat).
SFSG (Soy-Fortified Sorghum Grits)	1.5/360	16	15	
SFF1 12 % (Soy-Fortified Flour 12 %)	1.5/360	16	15–20	
SFRO (Soy-Fortified Rolled Oats)	1.6/370	21	5	
Incaparina (Central America)	1.6/370	28	5–10	
Balahar (India)	1.5/360	22	5–10	
Other blends				
SEF (supplement-enriched food: wheat, FPC, DSM, sugar)	1.7/400	20	5	Keep well for about 9 months.
Semper I (cereals, DSM, FPC, oil)	2.0/480	15	Fully precooked	
Milks and fish-protein concentrates				
DSM (Dried skim milk)	1.5/350	35		Milks have a high lactose content. DSM contains no vitamins A or D, unless this is mentioned on the bag. Milks provided by UNICEF, USA and Canada are usually enriched.
DFCM (Dried full-cream milk or whole milk)	2.1/500	25		
Sweetened condensed milk	1.3/320	13	Fully precooked	DFCM does not store well once a container has been opened (rancidity).
FPC (fish-protein concentrate)				FPC type A does not smell or taste of fish but is more expensive than type B.
type A	1.5/360	75		
type B	1.4/340	65		
Cereals				
Bulgur wheat (whole grain)	1.5/350	11	20 (less, if soaked overnight)	

[a] Values in MJ rounded to one decimal place on conversion from kcal_th.

Some foods sent as emergency relief are inappropriate for cultural reasons (religion, food habits, etc.), or because of unsuitable packaging (e.g., 95 % of the weight of the small bottles of vegetable mash for infants is made up of water and glass) or low nutritional value (sweets, luxury foods, etc.). Do not waste fuel and effort in distributing food containing only minute amounts of proteins and calories. Give it away to a local institution. If it is not acceptable, return or destroy it. Always inform your supervisors and the donor's local representative if donated supplies are inappropriate. This will help to improve the quality of later consignments.

Nutrient content of some commonly used special foods

The composition of special foods, as indicated in Table 4, varies with the availability and cost of the ingredients. However, the nutrient content remains *approximately* constant. All cereal-based formulas have a variable protein content, and the values shown are the lowest which occur.

Dried skim milk (DSM) is used as a high-quality protein source in most formulas. When only small amounts of milk (e.g., 50 g of DSM) are given daily, lactose intolerance will *not* be a significant problem among the general population.

Vitamins and minerals are usually added to most (but not all) processed foods so that 100 g of dry product meet the daily recommended allowance. DSM contains no vitamins A–D unless they have been added during processing (a measure increasingly adopted by supplying countries).

Whole cereals (e.g., bulgur wheat and SF bul) retain a high amount of B vitamins (e.g., thiamine).

Most processed foods are partially precooked, some are *fully* precooked and are called instant or ready-to-mix foods (DSM, DFCM, instant CSM, Semper I, etc.). Fully precooked foods are very convenient (since they can be cold-mixed) but they must be made up freshly *each time they are served,* especially if they are made up with unboiled water. Germs do multiply very quickly (within one to two hours) in a cold mixture of instant food and water, since there they find everything they need—water, sugar, proteins, etc.—at an ideal temperature. A food mixture contaminated by unsafe water becomes after a while much more dangerous than the water itself.

Instant foods must be: prepared just before meal-time with boiled water

or added to a porridge (gruel, etc.) after its preparation

or eaten in a dry form (DSM, FPC, etc.)

or added to the normal diet (e.g., to soup).

To facilitate identification of the contents of the food bags, once they are piled up in the warehouse, a special colour code was recently devised. Red is used for soy-fortified foods and blue for other commodities. The most usual symbols (printed on the sides of the bags) are as follows:

CORN-SOY MILK (CSM)	◆	← Red
INSTANT CORN-SOY MILK [1]	⧖	← Red
WHEAT–SOY BLEND (WSB) [1]	⬡	← Red
CORN MEAL	○	← Blue
SOY-FORTIFIED CORN MEAL	●	← Red
SOY-FORTIFIED FLOUR 6 %	✕	← Red
SOY FLOUR (TOASTED, DEFATTED)	♧	← Blue
SOY-FORTIFIED FLOUR 12 %	♣	← Red
ROLLED OATS (OATMEAL)	▢	← Blue
SOY-FORTIFIED ROLLED OATS	▧	← Red

[1] Sweetened and flavoured Instant-CSM and WSB are sometimes donated; they are identified by distinct symbols.

Preparing special foods

Always try cooking a small sample yourself to make sure the recipe works.

Cereals

Bulgur wheat and SF bul are not in powder form but in cracked whole grains, precooked to reduce cooking time and increase storage stability.

Add sufficient water to cover the grains in the pot.
Soak for a few hours (overnight).
Boil the cereals in the same water (B vitamins are present in this water) for 10–15 min (20, if no soaking).
Do not wash or rinse the grains after cooking.
If the cereal is not cooked long enough, it is poorly digested by children.
Pound finely (mash) for young children.
Proportions are about 1 part bulgur, 2 or 3 parts water. The volume more than doubles in cooking.

The same principles apply to most locally grown cereals.

Special blends (in powder form)

1. First mix one part of CSM or other blends with two parts of water (it is important, always to use *cold* water). *Slowly* add the special blend to the water *while stirring.* If the mixture is lumpy, continue stirring until it is smooth.
   To use in *porridge* form, pour the smooth mixture into an extra part of water. Boil for 8–10 min, stirring all the time. The porridge should be thick to provide enough proteins and energy per portion.
   To enrich the usual meal, add the smooth mixture. Keep cooking and boiling (while stirring) for 5–8 minutes.
2. CSM and other blends can be used as dry ingredients partially replacing cereal flours in almost every local dish (breads, tortillas, chapatis, etc.). Depending on local cereal availability and acceptability, the proportion can vary from 20% to 50%. Try locally with a sample (mixture time, as well as oil and water content, should sometimes be increased).
3. Instant foods, e.g., instant CSM, can be added to *cold boiled* water and served immediately without cooking.
4. Whenever possible add 30–40 g of edible oil per 100 g of the *dry* blend to increase the energy content. Mix and stir thoroughly. The mixture (dry blend plus oil) can be stored for a few days in a dry place. After addition of water and cooking, consume within a few hours.

Dried milks (DSM, DFCM)

Reconstitute milk with one part of dry milk to 4 parts of water.

First take a small amount of *cold water* (1–2 parts), then slowly add DSM or DFCM and keep stirring until the solution is smooth. Add the remainder of the water (boil for 3–5 min if it is contaminated). If the DSM is in bulk, add milk powder to boiled cold water and whisk until powder is well dissolved.
Dried milk can be added directly to porridge during preparation or before serving. Stir well.

Dried skim milk (6 parts), oil (2 parts) and sugar (1 part) can be mixed together and stored for up to one week; 1 part of the mixture added to 4 parts of water gives a high-energy liquid food with 0.42 MJ (100 kcal$_{th}$) and about 4 g protein per 100 ml (see also Chapter 5).

Concentrated or condensed sweetened milk

The milk should be diluted because of the high sugar content (43%). Protein should be added because of the low content after dilution.

Use the tin as a measure.   Mix three tins of water to the contents of one tin of concentrated sweetened milk.   For a standard size tin (content 400 g) add 30 g of dry skim milk (three full teaspoons) to half a can of water.   Mix together and stir well.   Boil for 3 min if the water is not safe.   The final preparation (1350 ml) contains 0.48 MJ (115 kcal$_{th}$), 4.5 g protein, and 2.4 g fat per 100 ml and should be served without delay.

Condensed milk should not be confused with evaporated milk (unsweetened) which can be reconstituted by adding boiled water.

Fish-protein concentrates (FPC)

These can be added to traditional dishes or consumed without any preparation, even by infants.   When accepted, they are a high-quality source of protein.

7. Communicable diseases: surveillance and treatment, immunization and sanitation

Surveillance of communicable diseases must be carried out as part of nutritional surveillance.

Treatment of the major acute diseases should be standardized.

Avoid expensive symptomatic treatment.

Prevention and treatment of dehydration in diarrhoeal diseases are the most important curative measures.

Drugs must be limited to a few basic items.

Food distributions may provide a good opportunity to immunize population groups. Mass measles immunization should be considered, wherever a cold chain (adequate refrigeration) can be maintained.

The provision of adequate latrines, a water supply, and washing facilities is a basic requirement in any camp. It is as important as the provision of basic medical care.

There is a close association between infectious disease and malnutrition, and the provision of basic medical care is an important part of a nutritional relief programme.

Where people are suffering badly from the effects of a food shortage, the provision of food is the first priority. Daily activities in the rural health services should be temporarily reoriented towards nutrition.

In most emergencies, some 75–90% of patients present with minor ailments (aches, pains, etc.). These patients divert medical attention and resources and should not be treated during emergencies.

Medical responsibility lies with the local health authorities. Expatriate medical relief workers should adapt themselves to local standards and procedures. Familiarity with the local culture, pattern of disease, and organization of medical services is as important as an advanced knowledge of medicine and medical techniques.

Surveillance

The surveillance of communicable diseases must be conducted as part of nutritional surveillance (Chapter 3). In addition to PEM, there are a number of important conditions that should be recorded regularly by dispensaries, clinics, maternal and child health centres, health workers, and field teams.

At the local level, symptoms suggestive of a disease should be recorded and reported even if the diagnosis is uncertain. For instance: fever without cough (malaria in endemic areas); diarrhoea (gastroenteritis, dysentry, severe diarrhoea with dehydration); cough with fever (respiratory infections—possibly tuberculosis, if lasting more than 2 weeks). The selection should be limited to diseases of major public health importance that are easy to treat or prevent.

Reports should give the age and sex of patients. No information (blank) is not equivalent to no disease. The presence and absence of disease must be reported clearly in order to differentiate between lack of information and negative reporting (no cases).

Treatment of the most important diseases during emergencies

The following guidelines may be used wherever no standardized treatment scheme is recommended by the national health services.

When qualified personnel are scarce, patients cannot be given individual attention by a physician. A *standard* treatment should be given for the disease most likely to cause the patient's symptoms (presumptive treatment). For instance, in an area where malaria is common, any person with fever for which there is no obvious cause (abscess, respiratory infection, etc.) should be treated for malaria.

— Wherever possible, use single-dose treatments and avoid giving a patient a large supply of tablets.

— Do not give mixtures of tablets. One drug is usually sufficient.

— Injections are very useful and often appreciated by patients. They are sometimes dangerous and almost always relatively expensive. Do not overuse them.

— Syrups and sugar-coated pills are no more active than tablets. Their use should be avoided since they may be 5–10 times as expensive.

TABLE 5. THE MOST IMPORTANT DRUGS DURING NUTRITIONAL EMERGENCIES a, b

Drug	Patients' age, height, average weight — Dosage				Frequency (divide total dose as shown in this column)
	under 1 year, under 75 cm, 5 kg	1–4 years, 110 cm, 10 kg	5–9 years, 110–140 cm, 15 kg	over 10 years, over 140 cm, 45 kg	
procaine penicillin in oil c	0.8 ml	1.6 ml	2.5 ml	3.3 ml	1 dose × 5 days
benzathine benzylpenicillin c	180 mg	360 mg	450 mg	600 mg	single dose
tetracycline capsules, 250 mg d	250 mg	500 mg	750 mg	1 000 mg	4 divided doses × 3–5 days (no more than 5 days to children under 6)
chloramphenicol capsules, 250-mg injections	250 mg / 250 mg	500 mg / 500 mg	1 g / 1 g	2 g / 2 g	4 divided doses × 3–5 days / 4 divided doses × 3–5 days
sulfonamide, 500-mg tablets (sulfadiazine + sulfamerazine + sulfadimidine)	750 mg	1.5 g	3 g	4.5 g	4 divided doses × 3–5 days
chloroquine (base) 100-, 150-, 300-mg tablets					
treatment	75 mg	150 mg	300 mg	450 mg	single dose
weekly prophylaxis	50 mg	100 mg	200 mg	300 mg	1 dose every week
bephenium hydroxynaphthoate (Alcopar) 5-g sachet	—	2.5 g	5 g	5 g	single dose (can be combined with tetrachloroethylene)
piperazine 500-mg tablets	1 g	2 g	4 g	4 g	single dose × 2 consecutive days
tetrachloroethylene	0.5 ml	1 ml	1.5 ml	2 ml	two divided doses, 1 day
tiabendazole (Mintezol)	250 mg	500 mg	750 mg	2 g	two divided doses × 2 days
benzyl benzoate 25 % (or DDT 10 % or BHC 2 %)	—	—	—	—	local application, 1 day; repeat if necessary
acetylsalicylic acid, 500-mg tablets (aspirin tablets) e	150 mg	500 mg	750 mg	1 g	2–4 divided doses
1 % tetracycline ophthalmic ointment (Achromycin)	—	—	—	—	local application to the eye 1–3 times a day

a Iron, vitamins, etc., should be added to the list according to the specific deficiencies in the area.
b Oral and intravenous rehydration fluids are mentioned earlier.
c Doses of penicillin can be considerably increased if necessary. Aqueous injectable penicillin and oral penicillin are less convenient and should be administered at 6-hourly intervals.
d Avoid repeated courses of tetracycline in children under 8 years, as these may cause discoloration of the teeth.
e Aspirin overdoses are very dangerous for infants.

The number of drugs required is small. Often about 20 major drugs are sufficient for the most common diseases encountered in rural areas. Expatriate doctors and hospitals must not request expensive modern drugs. Table 5 lists some of the most useful drugs with daily recommended dose and duration of treatment. According to the local situation, other drugs can be added to the list.

Moderate diarrhoea without dehydration

Malnourished children get diarrhoea easily, and diarrhoea makes malnutrition worse. Children with diarrhoea must drink a lot. Dehydration is the major risk. Give a solution containing salt and sugar (*by mouth*). A glucose-salt standard solution is used for prevention as well as for the treatment of mild dehydration. In one litre of boiled cooled water:

sodium chloride (table salt)	3.5 g	(1 level teaspoon)[1]
glucose (or if not available: table sugar)	20.0 g	(8 level teaspoon)[1]
sodium bicarbonate (baking soda)	2.5 g	(1/2 level teaspoon)[1]
potassium chloride	1.5 g	(1/2 level teaspoon)[1]

The ingredients are commercially available in aluminium foil or polyethylene bags (e.g., UNICEF "oral rehydration salts"). If necessary, they can also be prepared locally in the dispensary. The products need not be chemically pure. Use cooled, boiled water, but do not boil the final solution. If sodium bicarbonate and potassium chloride are not available, give a solution with only salt and table sugar. For doses, see guide to rehydration in Table 7. Antibiotics should not be given in cases of moderate diarrhoea unless there is blood or mucus in the stools. *Very important:* a child with diarrhoea must continue to get food. If blood or mucus is present in the stools, the child should be brought back to the health services.

Diarrhoea with dehydration

The child usually dies from dehydration, not from the infectious process. *Adequate treatment of the dehydration is the life-saving measure.* Table 6 is a guide to whether dehydration is mild or severe; Table 7 is a guide to rehydration. If there has been blood or mucus in the stools for 2 days, antibiotics can be given for 5 days—tetracycline, sulfonamides, or chloramphenicol (see Table 5). Consult national authorities on the recommended standard treatment for diarrhoea.

---

[1] The equivalents in "teaspoons" are, of course, very rough and ready, since teaspoons vary so much in capacity and the density and volume of the ingredients also vary considerably from batch to batch.

[2] For further details on rehydration, see: WORLD HEALTH ORGANIZATION. *Treatment and prevention of dehydration in diarrhoeal diseases.* Geneva, 1976.

TABLE 6. HOW TO DECIDE WHETHER DEHYDRATION IS MILD OR SEVERE [a]

Sign	Degree of dehydration	
	Mild	Severe
(1) Patient's appearance	Alert or restless Thirsty	Limp or unconscious Too weak to drink well or to drink at all Cold skin (shock)
(2) Skin elasticity	Normal or slightly less than normal	Poor
(3) Radial pulse	Present	Weak or absent
(4) Eyes, fontanelle	Normal or slightly sunken	Sunken
(5) Urine flow (difficult to tell in children)	Usually normal	Little or none
(6) Acute weight loss	Less than 5 %	More than 5 %

[a] Adapted from: World Health Organization, *Treatment and prevention of dehydration in diarrhoeal diseases.* Geneva, 1976.

TABLE 7. A GUIDE TO REHYDRATION [a]

Dehydration	What kind of fluid	How much to give	How quickly to give it
Mild:			
(a) Patients who can drink	glucose-salt oral solution (continue with breast-feeding)	encourage patients to drink continuously until they refuse	within 4–6 hours (usually given at home)
(b) Patients who need a nasogastric tube	glucose-salt oral solution	120 ml/kg body weight	6 hours
Severe:			
Patients who need intravenous fluid [b]	(a) Ringer's lactate or Hartman's solution (compound solution of sodium lactate)	100 ml/kg body weight	within 4–6 hours (or less in adults); half of the requirement to be given in the first hour [b]
	OR		
	(b) half-strength Darrow's solution (lactated potassic saline injection) with 2.5 % glucose (not so good for adults)	150 ml/kg body weight	6 hours (half of the requirement to be given in the first hour) [b]
	OR		
	(c) normal saline (if nothing else is available)	100 ml/kg body weight	6 hours (divided evenly) [b]

[a] Adapted from: World Health Organization, *Treatment and prevention of dehydration in diarrhoeal diseases.* Geneva, 1976.
[b] If given intraperitoneally, 70 ml/kg body weight can be given in 10–20 minutes instead of 4–6 hours.

The glucose-salt solution is given by mouth or with a nasogastric tube. Patients with severe dehydration and those who do not respond well to oral rehydration need intravenous fluids—either Ringer's lactate or Hartman's solution (compound solution of sodium lactate), or half-strength Darrow's solution (lactated potassium saline injection) with 2.5 % glucose. Normal saline is the poorest fluid, while glucose (dextrose) 5 % must not be used.

In emergency conditions, the fluids used for intravenous injection can be given intraperitoneally. This should be done by experienced health personnel:

Examine the abdomen carefully so as to avoid penetrating an enlarged liver, spleen, or bladder. Attach the sterile set to the bottle of sterile fluid, clean the skin, and push a 1.2-mm diameter (18-gauge) needle through the skin, just below the umbilicus. Then open the clamp on the tubing of the set and push the needle straight into the peritoneal cavity: when the peritoneal cavity has been reached, the liquid will flow in a steady stream. The full amount (70 ml/kg body weight) can be given in 10–20 minutes by allowing the fluid to flow as fast as possible. Remove the needle and place a dressing over the wound.

Do not give other drugs. Among the many medicines that are either no use or even dangerous in these emergency conditions are neomycin or streptomycin, purgatives, tincture of opium, paregoric or atropine, cardiotonics such as epinephrine or coramine, steroids, charcoal, kaolin, pectin, bismuth and Lomotil. Antibiotics need not be given unless there is blood or mucus in the stools or a definite clinical indication of bacterial infection.

Measles

Measles is usually easily diagnosed by the mother herself. The mortality is very high among malnourished children. The child must eat and drink even if he has no appetite, is vomiting, or has diarrhoea (taboos forbidding food for the sick child are not uncommon).

There is no specific treatment. If a severe cough develops (a slight cough is a normal part of the disease), this can be treated with an injection of long-acting penicillin. Watch for night blindness and xerosis: if in doubt, give 110 000 μg of water-miscible retinol palmitate (200 000 IU of vitamin A) intramuscularly. If a water-miscible preparation is not available, give the same amount orally in oil.

Malaria

In an area where malaria is common, all patients with fever should receive presumptive treatment against the disease; a single-dose treatment is used (see Table 5). If the fever does not subside within 12 hours of the first dose of chloroquine (and there is no possibility of chloroquine resistance), then the diagnosis is wrong.

Quinine injections are expensive and unnecessary unless there is local resistance to chloroquine. Chloroquine injections should as a rule be avoided.

Respiratory infections

The sick child must drink and eat to prevent malnutrition. Antibiotics should not be given in mild cases with slight fever and cough, but must be reserved for severe cases (penicillin or sulfonamides, preferably in combination, or tetracycline for 3 days). Long-acting penicillin injections are simplest since only one dose has to be given.

Tuberculosis

The disease must be treated for about one year, following the regimen used by the national tuberculosis programme. Do not initiate treatment unless it can be maintained for at least 6 months. The exception to this is in the case of severe PEM, since children who fail to respond to treatment with food for no apparent reason (e.g., diarrhoea, measles, etc.) may be suffering from tuberculosis, even though there are no clinical signs of the disease. The commencement of tuberculosis therapy may produce a rapid and dramatic nutritional improvement.

Cholera

Cholera causes sudden, severe diarrhoea with frequent watery stools. The treatment consists of correcting the dehydration; use the fluid described above, giving 50–70 ml/kg during the first hour and the same quantity during the next 3 hours. Patients who are severely dehydrated or cannot accept oral fluids must be rehydrated intravenously or through a nasogastric tube. Tetracycline may be given for three days.

Any suspected cases must be notified to the health authorities and, if possible, a sample of the stools (or a rectal swab) should be sent for laboratory examination. Strict quarantine is useless.

Scabies

The treatment consists in decrusting lesions with a 2 % copper sulfate solution and painting, under close supervision, all areas involved with DDT (10 %), BHC (2 %), or benzyl benzoate (20–25 %). Clothes should be boiled if possible and the whole family treated at the same time.

Worm infestations

Intestinal worms eat part of the child's food and contribute to malnutrition.

Two types of worm are particularly common:

1. *Ascaris (roundworms).* If the infestation is widespread, carry out mass treatment (all children) with piperazine citrate for 3 consecutive days.

2. *Hookworms.* If the infestation and anaemia are known to be common, give tetrachloroethylene, tiabendazole, or bephenium (safer but more expensive). If both hookworms and ascaris are present, treat first against ascariasis and then, on completion of the treatment, follow up with treatment for hookworm.

Immunization

Distributions of food to an otherwise scattered or nomadic population provide an excellent opportunity for improving the coverage of immunization campaigns.

Techniques

Doses and techniques differ with each vaccine and with each manufacturer. Follow the instructions of the manufacturer or the ministry of health.

● The use of a *jet injector* (Ped-O-Jet) can greatly increase the speed of immunization (500–600 shots/hour) and prevents the transmission of viral hepatitis and/or tetanus.

The children must be organized into orderly queues. The jet injector is most useful when several hundreds or thousands of children can be assembled for immunization at one session.

For each type of injection, a different nozzle is needed for the injector. Make sure that the appropriate nozzle is used before starting.

The person using the injector must be trained to perform maintenance and small repairs (this training should take only one day).

● If *needles and syringes* are used, do not use the same needle (or syringe) for more than one person, unless it has been sterilized. Hepatitis can be spread in this way but does not develop until 2–4 months later. Boiling the material for a few minutes is *not* enough to kill the hepatitis virus. When available, disposable plastic syringes are recommended.

Measles immunization

Vaccination against measles (a disease closely associated with PEM) is highly effective in giving long-term protection.

However, measles vaccine is probably the most difficult vaccine to use under field conditions, since it is extremely sensitive to heat (room temperature) and to sunlight. One hour after reconstitution of the freeze-dried vaccine, it can be almost completely inactivated without any visible change. In addition, it is rather expensive.

Mass campaigns are recommended *provided* a foolproof cold chain can be organized. This is usually possible in large refugee camps, but may be more difficult if the population is dispersed.

The vaccine must be:

— always kept cool (under 4oC, e.g., with ice) and protected from sun-light;

— reconstituted with *chilled* solvent and administered within one hour (destroy the partly used bottles at the end of the immunization ses-sion);

— administered *before* the seasonal outbreak of measles (do not vaccinate a camp or village because a severe outbreak has caused several deaths, since by then it is too late);

— administered to the age groups most likely to be victims of the next outbreak (where, for instance, measles usually affects children 2–3 years old, there is no point in immunizing those over 5 years old, most of whom will be naturally immunized);

— administered to severe cases of PEM before admission to a therapeutic feeding centre.

DPT (diphtheria, pertussis [whooping cough], and tetanus) immunization

Diphtheria, whooping cough, and tetanus are serious childhood diseases. Neonatal tetanus (resulting from umbilical infection) and whooping cough contribute to the very high mortality in the first year of life. Outbreaks of whooping cough can be common in refugee camps. Two to three doses of DPT vaccine must be given at suitable intervals of time to obtain a useful level of protection. The immunization of expectant mothers against tetanus (after 6 months of pregnancy) has a protective effect against umbilical tetanus of the newborn.

BCG (tuberculosis)

A good and long-lasting (at least 10 years) protection is obtained when an effective vaccine is administered by intradermal injection (use non-leaking Mantoux syringes used for tuberculin testing).[1]

Vaccinate all groups at risk regardless of tuberculin status (positive or negative). No screening is necessary.

BCG vaccine is sensitive to heat and sunlight. Always store the freeze-dried vaccine in a cool, dark place. Use the reconstituted vaccine immediately and do not expose the bottle to direct sunlight.

---

[1] UNIPAC catalogue number 07 865 00.

An ulcer develops at the site of BCG injection, resulting in a permanent scar. The population should be warned in advance that this is normal.

TAB (typhoid and paratyphoid vaccine)

Mass immunization against typhoid fever is not recommended in nutritional emergencies.

Cholera vaccine

This vaccine is not very effective. *Emergency* mass immunization should be discouraged.

Sanitation

Good sanitation is a basic requirement in any camp, but one which is usually ignored.

Detailed procedures are described in: ASSAR, M. *Guide to sanitation in natural disasters.* Geneva, World Health Organization, 1971.

Water supplies

Quantity and quality are both very important.

	Average daily consumption
Clinics, field hospitals	40–60 litres per person
Feeding centres	20–30 litres per person
Camps	15–20 litres per person

Sources of water vary so widely in quality and type that it is difficult to lay down general rules, but:

— where a single exposed source is being used for drinking-water, protect it from contamination, e.g., fence-in the area (radius 55 m) except at one point and employ a guard;

— where all available water is known to be contaminated it may be possible to provide clean drinking-water separately, e.g., brought in drums or by tanker from somewhere else;

— if it is likely that an emergency will continue for a long time, explore other solutions as soon as possible (piping, pumping and filtration equipment, bore holes or artesian wells)—discuss this with government or aid officials; funding and equipment may be available.

Water can be made safer by boiling it for 3–5 minutes or by chemical treatment. Chlorine and chlorine-liberating compounds are the most common disinfectants. They are available in several forms:

— bleaching powder (25 % by weight of available chlorine when fresh), deteriorates quickly when stored in humid and warm places;

— calcium hypochlorite, more stable, contains 70 % by weight of available chlorine;

— sodium hypochlorite, usually sold as a solution of approximately 5 % strength;

— chlorine tablets.

The dose of chlorine must be carefully determined (for example: 50–100 mg of available chlorine per litre for 12 hours to disinfect wells and springs). Seek the advice of sanitation workers. When indiscriminately distributed to the population, the tablets are usually of very limited benefit and, if taken by mouth, can be dangerous.

Latrines

Latrines must be provided wherever large groups of people are living together. The most useful types are described below:

The shallow trench latrine is a trench dug with hand tools. The trench is 30 cm wide and 50–100 cm deep. The length depends on the number of users (3–3.5 m for every 100 people). The shallow trench lasts about 2–7 days, after which it is filled in and a new one is dug.

The deep trench latrine is intended for long-term camps (of several months' duration). The trench is 2–4 m deep and 75–90 cm wide. The length depends on the number of users (1 m for each place, 4–5 places for every 100 people). When digging deep trenches shoring is required, since trenches easily collapse. The top is covered by a fly-proof floor made of strong pieces of wood or bamboo, allowing a good (50 cm) overlap on each edge. The floor is plastered with mud leaving holes approximately 25 cm in diameter at intervals of a metre. Cover up with earth when the trench is filled to 30 cm below ground level.

The bore-hole latrine. Where the subsoil does not contain rocks, a hole (diameter 40 cm; depth 5–6 m) is made with the use of earth-augers. Plan one bore-hole for every 20 persons.

Septic tanks. Where trench latrines are impracticable (because of sandy or very wet soil), it may be necessary to provide drainage into septic tanks. There are normally gravity drained, and it is therefore necessary either to build an elevated platform for the latrines or to use suitably sloping terrain. Septic tanks are available in many countries at no great cost.[1] Installation is usually straightforward, but professional advice should be sought.

Wherever latrines are provided, they should be:

— easily accessible at night;

— cleaned at least daily (if necessary, full-time staff should be employed to do this, since people will not use filthy latrines);

— sited well away from sources of drinking-water (at least 30 m from any source and 1.5–3 m above the water table).

---

[1] A complete prefabricated latrine and septic tank system (using butyl rubber tanks) is marketed by Oxfam, 24 Banbury Road, Oxford, England.

Washing facilities

If good water supplies are available, washing presents no problem. When the number of water points is limited, the provision of a special washing facility will save water and make the collection of water by individuals easier. Such a facility can easily be constructed with readily available materials, e.g., pierced drums for showers, etc.

If necessary and possible, provide facilities for boiling clothes—e.g., drums, firewood, and a changing and drying area for people with only a single set of clothing. Boiling clothes may be useful in the control of body lice (in combination with the use of insecticides, e.g., DDT, gamma BHC)[1] or of scabies (in combination with these insecticides or with the application of a tropical solution).

Sanitation as well as basic medical care and immunization are essential components of any relief programme to deal with nutritional emergencies.

---

[1] Widespread use of DDT and gamma BHC has led in some areas to the development of resistance to them by some insects—e.g., bedbugs, headlice, bodylice. Malathion and carbaryl are effective alternatives.

8. Camp administration, transportation, and food storage

Relief programmes are doomed to failure if the administrative and operational aspects are poorly managed.

Camps must be properly administered. Auxiliary personnel should be recruited from the population assisted and receive fixed salaries or work on a clearly defined food-for-work basis. Key personnel should not be from the population assisted as they are likely to be subjected to heavy pressure.

Transportation needs careful planning and close supervision to reduce thefts, waste, etc. Local traditional transportation (e.g., animals) is often the cheapest and most reliable.

Foods are perishable. Storage at the local level should meet some minimum requirements. Of these, cleanliness of the store and up-to-date stock-cards are the most important.

In the past, relief efforts have been more seriously impaired by lack of proper management than by neglect or ignorance of nutritional principles or techniques.

Camp administration

The number of hired personnel should be restricted to a few essential posts:

— store keeper, food supervisor

— registry clerk (with helpers, depending on size of camp)

— camp supervisor (distributions, sanitation)

— guards (if security is not provided by the authorities) with fixed salaries and working hours.

The responsible personnel should live close to the camp in proper lodgings. They must be familiar with the habits of the people they are assisting and speak their language. The use of interpreters may lead to misunderstandings, especially between foreign volunteers and nationals, because they sometimes tend to put their own views into their interpretations. It is recommended that the key personnel not be recruited from the assisted group because they are likely to be subjected to strong pressure.

As far as possible, the other personnel needed (for distribution, cooking, etc.) should be recruited within the camp on a clearly defined food-for-work basis.

The office should have proper tables and chairs, registry book(s), and a map of the camp on the wall, with the different sectors marked. There should also be a chart, preferably a blackboard indicating the number of inhabitants for each sector, as a basis for programmes of all kinds. A clearly written list of the names of the staff is helpful for visitors.

There should be a sheltered porch for waiting visitors.

The office should be locked after working hours.

A camp committee helps to obtain cooperation with the administration. There should at least be a contact group, consisting of one or more people in each sector of the camp, to spread information about distributions, vaccinations, important visits, changes in programmes, etc.

Transportation

Foods are bulky. Their transportation is often the cause of bottlenecks in a relief operation.

- To provide a full dry ration for one week to 10 000 persons, 12 three-ton truckloads are necessary (i.e., some 36 000 kg).

- A 4-wheel vehicle can carry about 500 kg of food in addition to the team in charge of food distribution and surveillance. This is the daily requirement of 20 families (5 persons each) or one supplementary meal for 250 children.

- Medical officers and supervisors need adequate transportation on a full-time basis. No supervision is possible without transport.

- Under bad conditions at least one out of 10 vehicles will be immobilized at any time for maintenance or repair.

- Considerable delays due to bad weather, poor roads, and breakdowns are common.

Therefore:

- A *realistic* itinerary should be planned long in advance. It should be flexible—the unexpected is part of the daily routine during emergencies.

- Use local traditional transportation as much and as early as possible. It is cheap and reliable. A camel can cover an average of 15 km per day and carry 200 kg. A donkey can carry only half of that but can negotiate very difficult country. For short distances, bicycle delivery can be very valuable (load 50 kg) as maintenance is relatively simple.

FIG. 17. BILL OF LADING [a]

TO:				NO.:		
DATE:				FROM:		
				VEHICLE NO.:		

DESPATCHED			RECEIVED		
Commodity	Number of bags/ containers	Condition	Commodity	Number of bags/ containers	Condition

Warehouse	Transporter	Consignee
Despatched:	I acknowledge that the supplies listed above have been received for transportation to the designated address.	I certify that all the items listed, unless otherwise noted, have been received.
Date: Time:		
Warehouseman's signature and stamp:	Carrier's signature:	Consignee's signature:
....	....	....

[a] From: *Food emergency manual.* Rome, World Food Programme (new edition in preparation).

Close supervision will reduce thefts during transportation. Each consignment should be accompanied by a "bill of lading" (Fig. 17) in at least two copies, of which one is returned to the head storekeeper with the signature of the receiver after careful checking when unloading. Damage to bags should be reported on this form. This simple procedure can save much food, provided appropriate sanctions are taken when indicated.

Each vehicle should have a log-book recording mileage and fuel; this should be checked regularly to prevent unauthorized trips and fuel thefts.

Food storage

Foods are perishable. Careful storage can minimize waste.

(*a*) *Storage at local level* should meet the following requirements.

● A "rule of thumb" is that one ton of processed foods in bags occupies a volume of approximately 2 m³. The usable space of a store is at least 25 % less than the total volume.

● The store should have a good roof and be dry and well ventilated. Whenever possible, use modern buildings for storage.

● Bags must not lie directly on the floor. Use pallets (Fig. 18), boards, heavy branches, or bricks, or put a layer of clean dry polyethylene bags underneath.

● Keep products at least 40 cm from the wall and 10 cm from the floor.

● Keep damaged bags apart from undamaged bags (possibly in a separate area). Keep a reserve of good empty bags.

● Keep each product separately.

● Pile the bags two by two crosswise to permit ventilation. In this way, they are steadier and easier to count.

● To avoid difficulty in handling and to keep packages from falling, do not stack them too high.

FIG. 18. PALLET

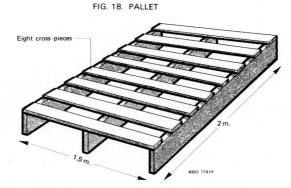

Eight cross-pieces

2 m.

1.5 m.

WHO 77819

Use boards 5 × 10 cm (on edge) for runners and strips 2.5 × 5 cm (laid flat) for crosspieces.

(*b*) *A close watch must be kept on food.*

● Limit access to the store to a few authorized persons.

● The key should stay with the storekeeper.

● Every item should have its own stock card (Fig. 19).

● The balance shown on the stock cards must be checked periodically by counting the actual number of items in stock.

● Food rotation is essential: the last food in should be the last to come out. Many items are marked with a date of manufacture. This date is often coded in the contract number on the bag. The local representative of the donor may help decode it.

FIG. 19. EXAMPLE OF STOCK CARD

CSM [a]

Bags (22.5 kg)

Date	Origin or destination	Received (in)	Distributed (out)	Balance (in stock)
10 May	From central store	32	—	32
12 May	To village A	—	10	22
13 May	From central store	27	—	49
″ ″	To mobile team	—	5	44
″ ″	To village B	—	7	37

[a] With locally bought food, the weight of bags might vary. The card then records kilograms rather than number of bags.

(c) Rats and vermin

Spilled foods or refuse attract rodents, insects and birds. The best method of control is to keep the food store clean. Store broken bags in a separate area and enclose the contents in a polyethylene bag. Keeping cats in the store helps to control rats.

Chemical control

Fumigation with methyl bromide or phosphine is a very effective way of killing rodents and insects in the store and vermin inside the bags. Fumigants are not expensive but may be toxic to human beings. If the manufacturer's instructions are carefully followed (dosage time, protection, etc.) the technique is safe and the food not impaired.

Poison baits are not very effective, especially if there is plenty of spilled food available.

Insecticides: spraying the store regularly with DDT or other products is an effective measure (the outer paper layer of most imported bags has already been impregnated with insecticides). Do not spray unless all bags are closed and the food is protected from direct contact with the insecticide.

(d) Disposal of spoiled foods

Particularly in tropical climates, it is almost inevitable that certain food items like cereals and dried fish get infested with vermin. People are often used to this, and the nutritional value of the foods is not changed and their safety may not be affected. Wet bags should be dried in the sun before being piled up and stored. Infested bags should be taken out and weevils sieved out. Distribute infested cereals or blends as soon as possible. Weevils or worms will float on water when the grains are soaked. Note that hard lumps in milk bags are harmless as long as there is no rancid smell.

Review of basic facts about food and nutrition

Nutrient requirements of humans

Nutrients

All foods are made up of five basic types of nutrient: carbohydrates, fats, proteins, vitamins, and minerals, in addition to variable amounts of water.

Carbohydrates

Carbohydrates are mostly starches and sugars of vegetable origin, being, for example, a major component of cereals and tubers. They are primarily a source of energy.

Fats and oils

Fats and oils are also a source of energy, having more than twice the energy content of carbohydrates and proteins. In most poor countries, most of the energy is derived from carbohydrate sources, especially cereals—fats accounting for a much smaller proportion.

Proteins

Proteins are body-building substances. Some proportion of protein is found in almost all human foods. Cereals, for example, contain about 8–12% protein. All proteins are composed of amino acids, of which some cannot be made by the body. These are called essential amino acids and must be obtained from food.

Proteins of animal origin contain all the essential amino acids in adequate amounts and are found in milk, meat, eggs, cheese, fish, and fowl.

Proteins of vegetable origin contain limited quantities of some of the essential amino acids. However, by combining different vegetable foods, e.g., cereals with legumes, or by adding some animal protein to vegetable sources, mixtures of higher quality can be obtained. It is possible for a human being to obtain an adequate quality of protein from mixed vegetable sources without eating protein from animal sources.

Vitamins

Vitamins are needed for the adequate functioning of the body. There are two main groups: first, *water-soluble vitamins*, e.g., the vitamin B complex—thiamine (B1), riboflavin (B2), and niacin—and vitamin C. Whole cereals, legumes, other vegetables, and animal foods are adequate sources of the B-complex vitamins. Vitamin C is found in raw fruits and vegetables. Vitamins A and D are examples of the other main group: *fat-soluble vitamins*. They are found in most animal products and significant amounts are stored in the body (liver, etc.). Vitamin A can also be formed in the body from pigments of yellow and green vegetables and fruits (carotenes) and vitamin D can be produced in the skin by exposure to sunlight.

Minerals

Iron is required for the formation of the red pigment in the blood (haemoglobin). Iron deficiency is a common cause of anaemia in many countries. Leafy vegetables, red meats, and fish are good sources of iron.

Sodium and potassium deficiency is only likely to be seen in individuals with profuse diarrhoea (see Chapter 8). Several other minerals are essential to the diet, but are not usually critical in emergency situations.

Water

Water is essential to sustain life. For practical purposes, water requirements may be considered to consist of the amount needed for replacement of the losses in faeces, urine, and transpiration. Young children are extremely vulnerable to dehydration (e.g., through profuse diarrhoea, vomiting, sweating).

The average minimum daily requirements of healthy children in warm climates are approximately as follows:

— at 1 month   400 ml
— at 4 months   600 ml
— at 12 months   800 ml
— at 3 years   1000 ml

Most infant foods, including milk, provide about 0.3 MJ (70 kcal$_{th}$)/100 ml and 95 % of their volume is water. When the energy content of food approaches 0.42 MJ (100 kcal$_{th}$)/100 ml, the water content is only 90 % of the volume of the food.

RECOMMENDED DAILY ENERGY AND PROTEIN INTAKES [a] FOR HEALTHY INDIVIDUALS

| Group | Energy MJ (kcal$_{th}$) | Protein (g) [b] | | Approximate proportion of the population in a developing country % |
		mixed diet with some animal protein	cereals possibly with legumes	
0–1 year	3.4 (820)	14 (breast-feeding) plus, after six months, weaning foods		3.0
1–3 years	5.7 (1 360)	21	27	9.0
4–6 years	7.7 (1 830)	25	33	8.7
7–9 years	9.2 (2 190)	29	37	8.5
10–14 years:				
males	11.7 (2 800)	46	58	6.3
females	10.3 (2 450)	40	50	6.2
Male adult (moderately active)	12.6 (3 000)	49	62	29.2
Female adult (moderately active)	9.2 (2 200)	39	48	26.2
Pregnancy (latter half)	10.7 (2 550)	49	63	1.5
Lactation	11.5 (2 750)	60	77	1.4
Average	9.2 (2 195)	37	47	—

[a] Adapted from *Handbook on human nutritional requirements*. Geneva, World Health Organization, 1974 (Monograph Series, No. 61).
[b] Adjusted to take digestibility and quality of protein into account.

Energy and protein intakes

The accompanying table shows the recommended energy and protein intakes for individuals of different ages or physiological status. The last column indicates the approximate proportion of the different groups in a developing country.

An adequate energy intake is the first priority when food is scarce.   Protein, carbohydrates, and fat supply energy at the following rate:

1 g carbohydrate provides approximately	0.017 MJ (4 kcal$_{th}$)
1 g fat provides approximately	0.038 MJ (9 kcal$_{th}$)
1 g protein provides approximately	0.017 MJ (4 kcal$_{th}$)

If an adequate energy supply is not provided, some protein will be burnt to provide energy and not used for body growth or repair, i.e., it will be used in the same way as carbohydrate or fat, which are much less expensive.

A part (20–40 %) of the energy requirement should be supplied from fats and oils, which greatly enhance the palatability of the diet, diminish its bulk (important for younger children), and reduce transport requirements.

Energy requirements vary widely even in normal individuals.   They are also increased by physical activity.   For example, a 65-kg man requires daily:

6.3 MJ (1500 kcal$_{th}$) when resting in bed day and night
11.3 MJ (2700 kcal$_{th}$) if lightly active in the daytime (clerk, office worker)
12.6 MJ (3000 kcal$_{th}$) if moderately active 8 hours a day
14.6 MJ (3500 kcal$_{th}$) if doing heavy work 8 hours a day (labourer)

Much higher intakes are required for the treatment of malnutrition.

Vulnerable groups

The energy and protein requirements of women are increased by pregnancy (+1.5 MJ (350 kcal$_{th}$) and +10–15 g protein/day) and lactation (+2.3 MJ (550 kcal$_{th}$) and +15–20 g protein/day) over and above their normal requirements.   The amount of proteins will vary with their quality.   Larger amounts of vegetable proteins are required.   Because of their rapid growth rate, young children require proportionally more energy and protein for each kg of body weight than adults do:

	MJ (kcal$_{th}$)/ kg body weight
infant	0.5 (120)
5 years old	0.4 (90)
11 years old	0.3 (70)
male adult	0.2 (45)

Pregnant women and young children are particularly likely to become malnourished in times of food shortage.   Young children are also more vulnerable to malnutrition for the following reasons:

● They require a greater number of feeds per day (3-4) than may be prepared for the family.

● They require more concentrated sources of energy and protein than may be supplied by available foods.

● Young children (between about 6 months and 5 years) are particularly subject to infections (measles, whooping cough, malaria, diarrhoea, etc.) which, by reducing appetite and increasing energy expenditure, may precipitate or worsen malnutrition.

● In some cultural contexts, adults are served first and younger children last.

Food given to sick children must not be reduced or restricted in quantity. On the contrary, they should receive additional food, whenever possible.

Foods and diets

Most diets in most countries contain adequate amounts of all the nutrients required for good health *if enough of the diet is taken to satisfy the individual's energy requirements.* This also applies to protein. Even a growing child, whose protein requirement is the highest (per unit of body weight) of any member of the population, if healthy, requires no more than 10% of his calories to be supplied from protein sources.

Commonly used foods (see Annex 2)

(*a*) *Cereal grains* (rice, corn, millet, sorghum, oats, and wheat)

These staple foods are the main source of energy (carbohydrates) and contain significant quantities of proteins (8–12%), vitamin B, and iron. Most vitamins (especially thiamine) are lost in the milling process. The whiter the flour, the greater the loss of vitamins, unless the flour is enriched or fortified with vitamins.

(*b*) *Legumes and oilseeds* (beans, peas, soya, groundnuts, etc.)

Legumes as a group contain about 20% of proteins (soy beans up to 40%), the B-complex vitamins, and iron. Legumes are particularly useful when eaten with cereals, as the proteins complement each other. They provide energy in a compact form but require careful storage because of their vulnerability to insects, rodents, and weevils. Digestibility can be increased by removing the skin after soaking overnight.

(*c*) *Tubers and roots* (yams, taro, cassava, sweet potato, potato, etc.)

Tubers and roots are the main sources of carbohydrates and are low in proteins (1–2%). Bulk and low protein content make them unsuitable as staple foods for infant feeding unless supplemented by foods richer in proteins.

(*d*) *Vegetables and fruits*

Vegetables and fruits are high in water and low in calories. They are often rich in provitamin A or carotenes, vitamins B and C, iron, and calcium, especially dark-green leafy vegetables (young cassava leaves, baobab leaves), which in addition have an appreciable protein content (2-4%).

(*e*) *Animal products* (meat, fish, milk and dairy products, eggs, etc.)

Of high protein quality, animal products are consumed in very small quantities in most developing countries in normal times and they may become even scarcer during emergencies. Small amounts add considerably to the quality and palatability of a diet. Local taboos might restrict their use in some groups (e.g., young children, pregnant women).

Milks are rich in protein, sugar, fat, calcium, and vitamins (except vitamin C, present only in human milk). All milks are poor in iron. Skim milk (non-fat milk) contains *no* fat-soluble vitamins A and D unless they have been added in the factory. It is important to check this on the label.

(f) Oils and fats

Oils and fats offer a compact source of calories. Fats derived from milk are sources of vitamin A and D, while vegetable fats contain no vitamin A and D, except for red palm oil which is extremely rich in carotenes.

(g) Human milk

This is the best and safest food for infants and young children (under 2 years). Breast-feeding should be promoted. Supplementary food must be given to the child at 4 months of age.

Bottle-feeding with commercial cow's milk preparations must be discouraged in areas with low standards of hygiene and maternal education, because of the high risk of fatal diarrhoeal disease in young infants.

Annex 2

Protein and energy content of some foods used in tropical countries [a]

(100-g edible portions, raw [b])

	Energy [c] MJ (kcal_th)	Proteins (g)	Waste (%) [d]
Cereals			
rice:			
lightly milled (brown)	1.5 (350)	7	0
overmilled (white or polished)	1.5 (350)	6	0
parboiled	1.5 (360)	7	0
maize, whole	1.5 (360)	9	0
millet and sorghum	1.5 (350)	10	0
wheat:			
bulgur wheat	1.5 (350)	11	0
whole wheat, soft	1.4 (340)	12	0
hard	1.4 (340)	11	0
wheat flour 80 % extraction rate	1.4 (330)	11	0
Vegetables and fruits			
cassava leaves, fresh	0.4 (90)	4	20 or more
sweet potato leaves, fresh	0.2 (50)	4	20 or more
dark-green leaves	0.2 (50)	2–5	20 or more
carrots, raw	0.2 (40)	1	10
tomato, fresh	0.1 (20)	1	2
citrus fruits (orange, lemon, lime, grapefruit, etc.)	0.2 (40)	0.5	25
mango, ripe	0.3 (60)	0.5	30–50
papaya, ripe	0.1 (30)	0.5	30
dates:			
raw	0.6 (140)	1	
dried	1.2 (290)	2	15
Fats and oils			
butter	2.8 (680)	—	0
ghee (butter oil)	3.6 (850)	—	0
palm oil	3.8 (900)	—	0
vegetable oils (others)	3.8 (900)	—	0

	Energy [c] MJ (kcal_th)	Proteins (g)	Waste (%) [d]
Legumes and oilseeds			
lentils	1.4 (340)	20	0
kidney beans	1.4 (330)	21	0
peas	1.4 (340)	25	0
chickpeas	1.5 (350)	20	0
black and red beans	1.5 (360)	25	0
nere (dried African locust bean)	1.7 (400)	32	—
groundnuts:			
whole, dried	2.3 (550)	23	30
press-cake	1.6 (380)	36	—
soya beans:			
dried seeds	1.7 (400)	33	0
partially defatted flour	1.1 (260)	46	0
Starchy roots and fruits, tubers			
cassava, fresh	0.6 (150)	1	15
flour	1.4 (340)	2	0
sweet potato, fresh, pale or orange	0.5 (110)	1	15
yam:			
tuber, fresh	0.5 (110)	2	15
flour	1.3 (320)	4	0
cocoyam	0.4 (102)	2	0
bananas:			
green	0.3 (70)	1	33
ripe	0.5 (120)	1	33
plantain bananas	0.5 (130)	1	33
breadfruit, pulp, fresh	0.4 (90)	1	25

[a] Adapted from FAO food composition tables and from: B.S. Platt: *Tables of representative values of foods commonly used in tropical countries*. London, HMSO, 1975 (Medical Research Council Special Report Series, No. 302).
[b] The content of cooked food varies depending on the method of cooking and especially the water content of the dish.
[c] Energy values in MJ have been rounded to one decimal figure when converting from kcalth.

Weight-for-height

A. YOUNG CHILDREN (BOTH SEXES)

Height (cm)	Weight (kg)				
	Standard	90 % standard	80 % standard	70 % standard	60 % standard
50	3.4	3.1	2.7	2.4	2.0
51	3.5	3.2	2.8	2.4	2.1
52	3.7	3.3	3.0	2.6	2.2
53	3.9	3.5	3.1	2.7	2.3
54	4.1	3.7	3.3	2.9	2.5
55	4.3	3.9	3.4	3.0	2.6
56	4.6	4.1	3.7	3.2	2.8
57	4.8	4.3	3.8	3.4	2.9
58	5.1	4.6	4.1	3.6	3.1
59	5.3	4.8	4.2	3.7	3.2
60	5.6	5.0	4.5	3.9	3.4
61	5.9	5.3	4.7	4.1	3.5
62	6.2	5.6	5.0	4.3	3.7
63	6.5	5.8	5.2	4.6	3.9
64	6.7	6.0	5.4	4.7	4.0
65	7.0	6.3	5.6	4.9	4.2
66	7.3	6.6	5.8	5.1	4.4
67	7.6	6.8	6.1	5.3	4.6
68	7.9	7.1	6.3	5.5	4.7
69	8.2	7.4	6.6	5.7	4.9
70	8.5	7.6	6.8	6.0	5.1
71	8.7	7.8	7.0	6.1	5.2
72	9.0	8.1	7.2	6.3	5.4
73	9.2	8.3	7.4	6.4	5.5
74	9.5	8.6	7.6	6.6	5.7
75	9.7	8.7	7.8	6.8	5.8
76	9.9	8.9	7.9	6.9	5.9
77	10.1	9.1	8.1	7.1	6.1
78	10.4	9.4	8.3	7.3	6.2
79	10.6	9.5	8.5	7.4	6.4
80	10.8	9.7	8.6	7.6	6.5
81	11.0	9.9	8.8	7.7	6.6
82	11.2	10.1	9.0	7.8	6.7
83	11.4	10.3	9.1	8.0	6.8
84	11.5	10.4	9.2	8.0	6.9
85	11.7	10.5	9.4	8.2	7.0
86	11.9	10.7	9.5	8.3	7.1
87	12.1	10.9	9.7	8.5	7.3
88	12.3	11.1	9.8	8.6	7.4
89	12.6	11.3	10.1	8.8	7.6
90	12.8	11.5	10.2	9.0	7.7
91	13.0	11.7	10.4	9.1	7.8
92	13.2	11.9	10.6	9.2	7.9
93	13.5	12.2	10.8	9.4	8.1
94	13.7	12.3	11.0	9.6	8.2
95	14.2	12.8	11.4	9.9	8.5
96	14.5	13.0	11.6	10.2	8.7
97	14.8	13.3	11.8	10.4	8.9
98	15.0	13.5	12.0	10.5	9.0
99	15.3	13.8	12.2	10.7	9.2
100	15.5	14.0	12.4	10.8	9.3
101	15.8	14.2	12.6	11.1	9.5
102	16.1	14.4	12.9	11.3	9.7
103	16.4	14.8	13.1	11.5	9.8
104	16.7	15.0	13.4	11.7	10.0
105	16.9	15.2	13.5	11.8	10.1
106	17.2	15.4	13.8	12.0	10.3
107	17.5	15.8	14.0	12.2	10.5
108	17.8	16.0	14.2	12.5	10.7
109	18.2	16.4	14.6	12.7	10.9

B. ADULTS [a]

Height (cm)	Males (weight in kg)				Female (weight in kg)			
	Standard weight	80 % standard	70 % standard	60 % standard	Standard weight	80 % standard	70 % standard	60 % standard
140					44.9	36.0	31.5	27.0
141					45.4	36.4	31.8	27.3
142					45.9	36.8	32.2	27.6
143					46.4	37.2	32.5	27.9
144					47.0	37.6	32.9	28.2
145	51.9	41.6	36.4	31.2	47.5	38.0	33.3	28.5
146	52.4	42.0	36.7	31.5	48.0	38.4	33.6	28.8
147	52.9	42.4	37.1	31.8	48.6	38.9	34.0	29.2
148	53.5	42.8	37.5	32.1	49.2	39.4	34.5	29.6
149	54.0	43.2	37.8	32.4	49.8	39.9	34.9	29.9
150	54.5	43.6	38.2	32.7	50.4	40.4	35.3	30.3
151	55.0	44.0	38.5	33.0	51.0	40.8	35.7	30.6
152	55.6	44.5	39.0	33.4	51.5	41.2	36.1	30.9
153	56.1	44.9	39.3	33.7	52.0	41.6	36.4	31.2
154	56.6	45.3	39.7	34.0	52.5	42.0	36.8	31.5
155	57.2	45.8	40.1	34.4	53.1	42.5	37.2	31.9
156	57.9	46.4	40.6	34.8	53.7	43.0	37.6	32.2
157	58.6	46.9	41.1	35.2	54.3	43.5	38.0	32.6
158	59.3	47.5	41.5	35.6	54.9	44.0	38.5	33.0
159	59.9	48.0	42.0	36.0	55.5	44.4	38.9	33.3
160	60.5	48.4	42.4	36.3	56.2	45.0	39.4	33.8
161	61.1	48.9	42.8	36.7	56.9	45.6	39.9	34.2
162	61.7	49.4	43.2	37.0	57.6	46.1	40.4	34.6
163	62.3	49.9	43.6	37.4	58.3	46.7	40.8	35.0
164	62.9	50.4	44.1	37.8	58.9	47.2	41.3	35.4
165	63.5	50.8	44.5	38.1	59.5	47.6	41.7	35.7
166	64.0	51.2	44.8	38.4	60.1	48.1	42.1	36.1
167	64.6	51.7	45.3	38.8	60.7	48.6	42.5	36.4
168	65.2	52.2	45.7	39.2	61.4	49.2	43.0	36.9
169	65.9	52.8	46.2	39.6	62.1	49.7	43.5	37.3
170	66.6	53.3	46.6	40.0				
171	67.3	53.9	47.1	40.4				
172	68.0	54.4	47.6	40.8				
173	68.7	55.0	48.1	41.2				
174	69.4	55.6	48.6	41.7				
175	70.1	56.1	49.1	42.1				
176	70.8	56.7	49.6	42.5				
177	71.6	57.3	50.2	43.0				
178	72.4	58.0	50.7	43.5				
179	73.3	58.7	51.3	44.0				

[a] Based on: JELLIFFE, D.B. *The assessment of the nutritional status of the community.* Geneva, World Health Organization, 1966 (Monograph Series No. 33), pp. 238–241.

C. ALTERNATIVE THRESHOLDS OF MALNUTRITION USING THE REFERENCE VALUE (MEDIAN)
LESS TWO AND THREE STANDARD DEVIATIONS (CHILDREN, BOTH SEXES) [a]

Height (cm)	Reference weight (kg)	Standard deviation SD	Threshold of malnutrition	
			Less 2 SD	Less 3 SD
50	3.4	0.38	2.6	2.3
51	3.5	0.41	2.7	2.3
52	3.7	0.44	2.8	2.4
53	3.9	0.47	2.9	2.5
54	4.1	0.50	3.1	2.6
55	4.3	0.52	3.3	2.7
56	4.6	0.54	3.5	3.0
57	4.8	0.57	3.7	3.1
58	5.1	0.59	3.9	3.3
59	5.3	0.61	4.1	3.5
60	5.6	0.63	4.3	3.7
61	5.9	0.65	4.6	4.0
62	6.2	0.66	4.8	4.2
63	6.5	0.68	5.1	4.5
64	6.7	0.70	5.4	4.6
65	7.0	0.71	5.6	4.9
66	7.3	0.72	5.9	5.1
67	7.6	0.74	6.1	5.4
68	7.9	0.75	6.4	5.6
69	8.2	0.76	6.7	5.9
70	8.5	0.77	6.9	6.2
71	8.7	0.79	7.2	6.3
72	9.0	0.80	7.4	6.6
73	9.2	0.81	7.6	6.8
74	9.5	0.82	7.8	7.0
75	9.7	0.83	8.1	7.2
76	9.9	0.84	8.3	7.4
77	10.1	0.84	8.5	7.6
78	10.4	0.85	8.6	7.8
79	10.6	0.86	8.8	8.0
80	10.8	0.87	9.0	8.2
81	11.0	0.88	9.2	8.4
82	11.2	0.89	9.4	8.5
83	11.4	0.90	9.6	8.7
84	11.5	0.91	9.7	8.8
85	11.7	0.92	9.9	8.9
86	11.9	0.92	10.1	9.1
87	12.1	0.93	10.3	9.3
88	12.3	0.94	10.5	9.5
89	12.6	0.95	10.7	9.7
90	12.8	0.96	10.8	9.9
91	13.0	0.97	11.1	10.1
92	13.2	0.98	11.3	10.3
93	13.5	1.00	11.5	10.5
94	13.7	1.01	11.7	10.7
95	14.2	1.24	11.8	10.7 [b]
96	14.5	1.27	12.0	10.7
97	14.8	1.29	12.2	10.9
98	15.0	1.32	12.4	11.0
99	15.3	1.34	12.6	11.3
100	15.5	1.37	12.8	11.4
101	15.8	1.39	13.0	11.6
102	16.1	1.42	13.3	11.8
103	16.4	1.44	13.5	12.1
104	16.7	1.46	13.7	12.3
105	16.9	1.49	14.0	12.4
106	17.2	1.51	14.2	12.7
107	17.5	1.54	14.5	12.9
108	17.8	1.56	14.7	13.1
109	18.2	1.58	15.0	13.5

[a] Waterlow et al. *Bull. World Health Organ.*, **55**: 489–498 (1977). Full tabulation available from Nutrition, World Health Organization, 1211 Geneva 27, Switzerland.
[b] Adjusted value.

Annex 4

Arm-circumference-for-height, young children (both sexes)

Height (cm)	Standard arm circumference (cm)	90 % standard	85 % standard	80 % standard	75 % standard	70 % standard	60 % standard
54	11.1	10.0	9.4	8.9	8.3	7.8	6.7
56	11.6	10.4	9.9	9.3	8.7	8.1	7.0
58	12.2	11.0	10.4	9.8	9.1	8.5	7.3
60	13.0	11.7	11.0	10.4	9.7	9.1	7.8
62	13.9	12.5	11.8	11.1	10.4	9.7	8.3
64	14.2	12.8	12.1	11.4	10.6	9.9	8.5
66	14.4	13.0	12.2	11.5	10.8	10.1	8.6
68	14.8	13.3	12.6	11.8	11.1	10.4	8.9
70	15.4	13.9	13.1	12.3	11.5	10.8	9.2
72	15.6	14.0	13.3	12.5	11.7	10.9	9.4
74	15.7	14.1	13.3	12.6	11.8	11.0	9.4
76	15.8	14.2	13.4	12.6	11.8	11.1	9.5
78	15.9	14.3	13.5	12.7	11.9	11.1	9.5
80	15.9	14.3	13.5	12.7	11.9	11.1	9.5
82	15.9	14.3	13.5	12.7	11.9	11.1	9.5
84	16.0	14.4	13.6	12.8	12.0	11.2	9.6
86	16.1	14.5	13.7	12.9	12.1	11.3	9.7
88	16.2	14.6	13.8	12.9	12.1	11.3	9.7
90	16.2	14.6	13.8	13.0	12.1	11.3	9.7
92	16.3	14.7	13.9	13.0	12.2	11.4	9.8
94	16.4	14.8	13.9	13.1	12.3	11.5	9.8
96	16.5	14.9	14.0	13.2	12.4	11.5	9.9
98	16.6	14.9	14.1	13.3	12.4	11.6	10.0
100	16.7	15.0	14.2	13.4	12.5	11.7	10.0
102	16.8	15.1	14.3	13.4	12.6	11.8	10.1
104	16.9	15.2	14.4	13.5	12.7	11.8	10.1
106	17.1	15.4	14.5	13.7	12.8	12.0	10.3
108	17.3	15.6	14.7	13.8	13.0	12.1	10.4
110	17.4	15.7	14.8	13.9	13.1	12.2	10.4
112	17.6	15.8	15.0	14.0	13.2	12.3	10.6
114	17.8	16.0	15.1	14.2	13.3	12.5	10.7

Annex 5

The QUAC stick[a]

Preparation of the QUAC stick (to measure arm-circumference-for-height)

1. Secure a straight pole about 140 cm long and 4 cm wide.
2. Smooth one surface to take marking by pen.
3. Select from the table overleaf two scales out of the three (85 %, 80 %, 75 %) and the corresponding height values listed.
4. Tape a centimetre rule to the stick so that it will not move during marking. Measuring from the bottom, make on the left a mark at each of the heights indicated on the higher scale selected (e.g., 85%) and on the right, another mark at each of the heights listed for the second scale selected (e.g., 80% or 75%).
5. Remove the taped centimetre rule.
6. Extend the height marks to either edge of the stick with clearly drawn lines (1.5 cm long) using different colours for each scale (left and right).
7. Using the table again, mark at the line for each height the arm-circumference figure corresponding to that height.

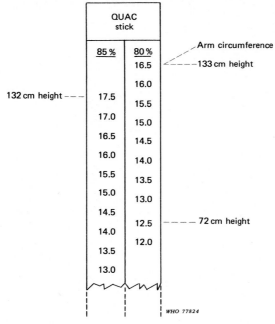

DIAGRAM OF QUAC STICK SHOWING 85% AND 80% ARM CIRCUMFERENCES FOR VARIOUS HEIGHTS

---

[a] Based on: ARNHOLD, R. *J. trop. Pediatr.*, **15**: 243 (1969); and DAVIS, L. E., *Am. J. Clin. Nutr.*, **24**: 358 (1971).

— 93 —

Use of the stick

After measuring the arm circumference, place the stick behind the child (standing up) and look for his arm-circumference value on the left-hand side. If the child's actual height is below the corresponding mark on the stick he is *not* malnourished according to the selected standard or scale (85% for instance). Conversely, if he is taller than the level on the stick at which his measured arm circumference is found, he is malnourished (under 85%, for instance). In this case, compare with the scale on the right-hand side.

BASIC DATA FOR THE MANUFACTURE OF THE QUAC STICK
(ARM-CIRCUMFERENCE-FOR-HEIGHT)

Height (cm)	AC 85 % (cm)	Height (cm)	AC 80 % (cm)	Height (cm)	AC 75 % (cm)
132	17.50	133	16.50	132 ½	15.50
129	17.00	129	16.00	129	15.00
126	16.50	125	15.50	125	14.50
122	16.00	121	15.00	122 ½	14.25
117 ½	15.50	118 ½	14.75	120	14.00
112	15.00	116	14.50	117 ½	13.75
109	14.75	114	14.25	116	13.50
106	14.50	112	14.00	113	13.25
101	14.25	107	13.75	108	13.00
96	14.00	104	13.50	105	12.75
88	13.75	98	13.25	100	12.50
80	13.50	92	13.00	92	12.25
72	13.25	82	12.75	84	12.00
		72	12.50	72	11.75

Random surveys and sampling techniques

In large population groups, measurements can be performed only on a sample. To draw any valid conclusion, the sample must be *representative* of the whole population. For instance, nutritional data obtained from health services are not representative of *all* the population. Nor are those collected in the most accessible villages or in camps that are reported to be in a bad state. Some randomization is essential.

The steps to take are as follows:

Definition of the objective of the survey. To estimate the nutritional status in camp A; to compare the nutritional status in villages A, B, C, and D; etc.

Definition of the population to be surveyed: Children; ethnic group; sedentaries and/or nomads; etc.

Obtaining the sample

● Obtain census data and a list of all settlements in the area (from ministries of statistics and planning or malaria control services). If these are unavailable, the population can be estimated by counting the dwellings and estimating the average number of people in each dwelling.

● Divide the population into groups that are similar with respect to the information to be collected. It is confusing if information from pastoral nomads cannot be separated from that obtained from sedentary subsistence farmers or urban settlers.

● Draw a random sample. Villages, camps, or other populations can be selected from the area at random for each defined group. At the village or camp level, households or families will be selected. Use random numbers as in Table A. [1]

— Number villages, camps, etc., consecutively in the list or on the map.

— Choose a first random number "at random" (e.g., shut your eyes and use a pin) then take every following number in the table to identify a sample point until the required number of sample points have been selected.

— Never change because a village selected is too remote or is close to a bigger or "more affected" place you feel should be surveyed in preference to the randomly selected "unimportant" village.

— Repeat the random process to select households and children at the level of the village.

● Determine the sample size: this depends on your objectives and need for accuracy. Seek professional advice.

---

[1] Please note that these numbers are given only as examples and those responsible for the sampling should use the more extensive table of random numbers in the publication by Fisher & Yates referred to in the note to Table A or similar tables in other statistical textbooks.

For instance, if the observed percentage of malnourished children from a sample of 100 children is 10%, the most one can say with a 95% chance of being right (probability level) is that the true (and unknown) proportion of malnourished children in the *total* child population is somewhere between 5% and 18% (confidence interval). Table B shows the respective confidence intervals at the 95% probability level for various sample sizes and observed percentages of malnutrition.

A. RANDOM NUMBERS [a]

76	58	30	83	64	87	29	25	58	84	86	50	60	00	25
47	56	91	29	34	05	87	31	06	95	12	45	57	09	09
10	80	21	38	84	90	56	35	03	09	43	12	74	49	14
00	95	01	31	76	17	16	29	56	63	38	78	94	49	81
07	28	37	07	61	11	16	36	27	03	78	86	72	04	95
20	26	36	31	62	68	69	86	95	44	84	95	48	46	45
31	56	34	19	09	79	57	92	36	59	14	93	87	81	40
98	40	07	17	81	22	45	44	84	11	24	62	20	42	31
24	33	45	77	58	80	45	67	93	82	75	70	16	08	24
01	31	60	10	39	53	58	47	70	93	85	81	56	39	38
50	78	13	69	36	37	68	53	37	31	71	26	35	03	71
90	78	50	05	62	77	79	13	57	44	59	60	10	39	66
46	72	60	18	77	55	66	12	62	11	08	99	55	64	57
47	21	61	88	32	27	80	30	21	60	10	92	35	36	12
12	73	73	99	12	49	99	57	94	82	96	88	57	17	91
23	54	20	86	85	23	86	66	99	07	36	37	34	92	09
65	76	36	95	90	18	48	27	45	68	27	23	65	30	72
37	55	85	78	78	01	48	41	19	10	35	19	54	07	73
87	12	49	03	60	41	15	20	76	27	50	47	02	29	16
83	05	83	38	96	73	70	66	81	90	30	56	10	48	59

[a] Taken from Table XXXIII of: Fisher, R. A. & Yates, F. *Statistical tables for biological, agricultural and medical research*, 6th ed., Longman Group Ltd, London, 1974 (previously published by Oliver & Boyd, Edinburgh) by permission of the authors and publishers.

B. CONFIDENCE INTERVALS AT 95% PROBABILITY LEVEL CORRESPONDING TO
VARIOUS SAMPLE SIZES AND SAMPLE PERCENTAGES

Sample size	Percentage observed in sample					
	5%	10%	20%	30%	40%	50%
30	1–18	2–26	8–39	15–49	23–59	31–69
40	1–17	3–24	9–36	17–47	25–57	34–66
50	1–15	3–22	10–34	18–45	26–55	36–65
60	1–14	4–20	11–32	19–43	28–54	37–63
80	1–12	4–19	12–31	20–41	29–52	39–61
100	2–11	5–18	13–29	21–40	30–50	40–60
200	2–9	6–15	15–26	24–37	33–47	43–57
300	3–8	7–14	16–25	25–36	35–46	44–56
400	3–8	7–13	16–24	26–35	35–45	45–55
500	3–7	8–13	17–24	26–34	36–45	46–55
1000	4–7	8–12	18–23	27–33	37–43	47–53
2000	4–6	9–11	18–22	28–32	38–42	48–52

A rough idea should be formed before the survey of the likely or expected proportion of malnourished children. This can be done by a very rapid and non-randomized survey of one or two villages thought to be representative of the area, using the same anthropometric technique and cut-off point to define malnutrition.

The sample size is determined by the degree of precision desired. If, for instance, the observed percentage of malnutrition is about 20%, a total sample size of 100 will make it possible to locate the *true* rate of malnutrition somewhere between 13% and 29%. If considerable accuracy is required, for instance 18–22%, a sample size of 2000 is necessary. Confidence intervals for simple random sampling are given in Table B.

The number of sites selected at random will vary with the total sample size and the observed percentage of malnutrition. As a general rule, it is essential that the total population sampled be distributed in a sufficient number of sites or clusters (at least 10) to assure the representativeness of the findings. At least 25 children should be examined in each site.

Very important. If you want to compare the results of the various clusters (sites, villages, camp), the sample size at each cluster (and not the total sample size) will determine the accuracy of the result. When cluster sampling is used, the confidence intervals for the same sample size may tend to be wider than those given in Table B. However, an increase in sample size to secure the same confidence interval with cluster sampling may not necessarily be more expensive.

● Do not draw far-reaching conclusions from small differences between two or more rates. These can be due to chance. Statistical tests are necessary. It is particularly important to reduce nonsampling errors (including bias). Seek professionnal advice.

Simple field test for vitamin A in dried skim milk

A simple field test has been developed to check the presence of vitamin A in dried skim milk (DSM). About 35 ml of trichloroacetic reagent are prepared by dissolving 50 g of crystalline reagent grade trichloroacetic acid in 5 ml of distilled water, preferably heated to about 60°C.[a] The resulting reagent is highly corrosive and irritating; it should never be pipetted by mouth and any drop that comes accidentally into contact with the skin, mouth, or eyes should be rinsed immediately and copiously with water. The reagent is light-sensitive and should be stored in the dark, preferably in a brown bottle, itself kept in some opaque container, box, or cupboard. The use of a freshly prepared solution appears advantageous. This seldom involves any difficulty as crystalline trichloroacetic acid is one of the most commonly used reagents in clinical and biochemical laboratories.

The test is carried out in two steps and requires one saucer and two glass or china cups. (1) Place a teaspoonful of DSM in the saucer and add a few drops of reagent; if the wet powder turns blue, vitamin A is present, but if there is no colour change, the test could be negative or false and should be checked. (2) To check, place 15 g of DSM in each cup, add 15 ml of water to the first, and stir, preferably with a glass or plastic rod or spoon, until a white slurry is produced. Then add 15 ml of reagent to the second cup and stir in the same way. If vitamin A is present, the colour will become pale blue or green in about one minute, quite distinct from the white slurry in the first cup. If vitamin A is absent, the slurries in both cups will look alike. To clean the utensils, they should be rinsed promptly,[b] thoroughly, and repeatedly with water. To render the reagent harmless before disposal, it should be diluted a hundredfold or more.

This qualitative test is designed for use under field conditions; it is not meant as a substitute for quantitative determinations.

---

[a] The laboratory that prepares the reagent may wish to supply convenient measuring spoons to handle 15 g of DSM and 15 ml of liquid: tolerances of ± 10% are of no consequence for the test, but account should be taken of the 30–40% density variations existing between batches of DSM.

[b] Delayed cleaning-up may be laborious.